A Picture of Health

COLLECTING PERSPECTIVES

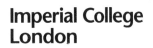

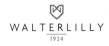

The contents of this book, as well as films indicated by the video symbol ▇◀ and additional images contributed to *A Picture of Health*, can be found at lms.mrc.ac.uk/picture-of-health.

Abbreviations
MRC   Medical Research Council
LMS   London Institute of Medical Sciences
UKRI   UK Research and Innovation
BPoD   Biomedical Picture of the Day

Published by MRC UKRI, Polaris House, Swindon SN2 1FL

British Library Cataloguing in Publication Data
A catalogue record for this book is available from the British Library

ISBN 978 1 3999 2784 0

Editors *Amanda Fisher, Kiki von Glasow, Lindsey Goff, Andree Molyneux*
Art direction and project management *Richard Adams Associates*
Website design *George Snow*
Design and technical assistance *Sam Adams* and *Red Dot*
Cover illustration *Jerry Yi Chang*, coloured pencils on paper
Printed by *Northend*, Sheffield

Foreword
SUSAN WATTS

Each Picture Tells a Story

We didn't know that a pandemic was just around the corner when our project *A Picture of Health* began. Nowadays, in the not-quite-post-pandemic world into which we launch this collection, we all pay a bit more attention to how we feel and how we relate to the world around us. This is a healthier way to live and, for each of us our 'picture' of health will be something unique.

It was this uniqueness that the team that coaxed this project into the world aimed to capture; we grappled with how best to ensure contributions from all walks of life, from bankers to writers from dancers to carers. We wanted to hear not just from the celebrated and the well-known, who already have a voice, but also from those less noticed and less loud. We especially wanted to hear from the people who keep our communities alive, the healthcare workers and the shopkeepers, the makers as well as the shakers. Most importantly, we wanted to hear from the voices of the communities that live and work close to the new building of the MRC London Institute of Medical Sciences (LMS), whose official launch this collection celebrates.

You will find all these voices gathered in this book. There are well known names from the worlds of science, finance, journalism and politics: from economist Mervyn King, who was Governor of the Bank of England during the financial crisis of 2007 to 2008 (p. 42), to plant biologist Ottoline Leyser, science leader and champion of equality, diversity, and inclusion (p. 12).

London, home to the LMS, is also well represented. There is a collection of poetry called *A Drop of Hope*, from the Francis Crick Institute, inspired by the words of those who received a COVID-19 vaccine at its King's Cross building. There is a photograph from Mayor Sadiq Khan, who celebrates the "energy, ideas and imagination" of the city's people. There are contributions too from those who work at the LMS, from the researchers and support staff at its home on the Hammersmith Campus near White City in West London.

You will find local characters such as Ronald 'Charlie' Phillips, nickname *Smokey*, a Jamaican-born restaurateur, photographer, and documenter of Black London; he is best known for photographs of Notting Hill during the migration from the Caribbean to London (p. 202). There's poetry too, with a fresh take on being a slug, from Suzanne Iwai; she describes herself as an autistic activist who has lived on the White City estate near the LMS for twenty years (p. 84). There's a touching drawing from the Wormwood Scrubs Pony Centre for those with special needs, by resident artist Romaine Dennistoun (p. 194).

Life resists categorisation
The collection is not structured, and is largely drawn from the skewed perspective of the UK with a small but significant group of contributions, some 15 percent, from further afield. These 'pictures' are as eclectic as their origins, which stretch from Australia to Bangladesh, The Gambia, Germany, Palestine, Spain, Tibet and the USA. Though wide in its reach, at this stage the collection is essentially compiled from an extended network of those colleagues, friends and acquaintances who felt moved to respond to our initial call for ideas. For someone like me, with a background in science journalism, I have found the process of building this collection somewhat meandering. I seek out order, and so a book without Contents runs against my nature. But then life is messy, unpredictable and resists categorisation. Sometimes it's good to hold back from imposing structure, and what has emerged here is something quietly beautiful.

My hope is that this is just the beginning, and that the project will develop to include more and more people from a wider and wider circle of backgrounds and experiences, reinforcing its relevance. The next phase will be online, in digital form, on the project's website lms.mrc.ac.uk/picture-of-health.

Each picture of health consists of an image and a brief descriptive text. This text can be read alone, without reference to the biography of the contributor, but the impact is greater if you read both. The summary text provides a glimpse of why the contributor sees their piece as

A Picture of Health, and the biography reveals a little of who they are and the life that has brought them to this point.

For me, an early contribution still best illustrates the project's essence. This comes from the curator of *A Picture of Health* Lindsey Goff. Lindsey edits another successful public engagement project from the LMS, called *Biomedical Picture of the Day* (BPoD) bpod.mrc.ac.uk. She sent in a photograph of her garden bench, adorned with a rich coating of *Usnea* 'beard' lichens. Their growth is possible because the bench sits in secluded moorland, where air pollution is minimal. She describes how these lichens are susceptible to sulphur dioxide and are extinct in many areas of the UK. She includes a hopeful note; that as we strive to protect clean air, through regulation of emissions and pursuit of cleaner energy, we may one day see lichen-rich benches in our towns and cities, as well as our countryside.

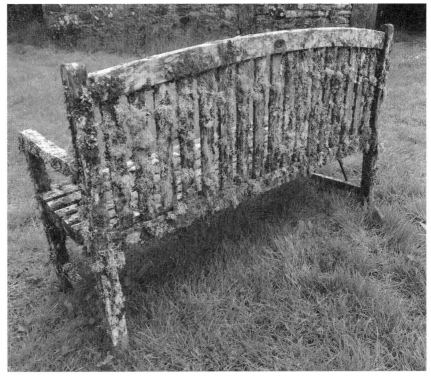

Lichen-covered garden bench on Dartmoor. Photograph: Lindsey Goff

Some contributors sent in their ideas before the pandemic. Most came after it had struck, and you can sense the pandemic's influence as a disrupter. Many personal and professional tragedies will have unfolded during this time, and the collection is shot through with themes heightened by the collective experience of the pandemic period; themes of sharp observation, of connection with others, and around the strength derived from belonging.

Observation

There is a cluster of contributions that delve into a world we have only been able to 'see' with evolving technologies. These celebrate imaging techniques that take us beyond the limits of our own eyes, providing insight beyond the obvious. Some of these techniques, such as the scans now commonplace in medical diagnostics, first came into use at the Hammersmith Hospital campus where the LMS is based.

Oliver Howes, professor of molecular psychiatry at King's and Imperial Colleges London, sent dramatic coloured images of the brain. These show that a brain with schizophrenia has less of a vital protein marker than does a healthy control. This deficiency limits communication between nerve cells, a picture of health that could help lead to treatments (p. 173). Particle physicist Frank Close describes the striking simplicity of an image of positron-electron annihilation. This is the basis of Positron Emission Tomography, or PET scanning, a medical technology that helps to save lives every day (p. 76). LMS scientist Karen Sarkisyan, sent in eerie images of bioluminescence in plants. His work could result in tissues and organisms that self-report their state of health, simply by glowing in the dark (p. 72).

Connection

Connection with others, and with place, is everywhere in these pages. Some of the shortest texts describe the most profound of human experiences. The poems here feel deeply personal: the haunting lines of Elisha Gabb evoke the soul-warming power of a pond's cold water (p. 98); and Brian Patten's ode to sharing a peach says much in so few words (p. 198). Photographic artist Celine Marchbank sent a picture of a squash flower from her allotment and describes the healing power of tending the plot after her mother's death: "It reminds me of her, and I feel connected. It is a happy place for me to be... It's my picture of health, every time I walk through the gates I feel well again" (p. 178).

Some contributors turn their gaze to the natural world and their lifelong connection to it. Nicholas Owens, executive director of the Scottish Association for Marine Science, sent a photograph of a happy whale...for him, the epitome of all that he loves about our oceans (p. 106). Patrick Vallance, the Government's Chief Scientific Adviser, sees beauty in hibiscus blooms in his garden, and a link with chemistry and the beginnings of the pharmaceutical industry (p. 211).

Belonging
Many contributions evoke family and community. Mervyn King's intimate reflection on support across generations conjures the feelings of hope that such connections can bring, as does Ottoline Leyser's carefree photograph of her niece flying a kite.

A photograph from table tennis coach Chris Beckley captures the spirit of "fun, laughter, creativity, friendship and community" that he shares with others through his passion for the sport.

Delight is palpable in the photograph submitted by Amanda Fisher, Head of the Institute of Clinical Sciences at Imperial College London, and originator of the project *A Picture of Health*. Her shot shows a sink full of used scientific glassware, which she says was a joyful sign of the return of busy scientific life as researchers came back to their labs after lockdown (p. 167). And it is the sense of purpose in joint venture that moves Robert Gallo, the scientist who co-discovered HIV as the cause of AIDS and developed the HIV blood test. His picture of health is not just the faded grey image of the 'Western blot' laboratory read-out that confirmed that HIV caused AIDS, but also a black and white photograph of his youthful lab group "passionate about their work and all in the prime of their life" from 1984 (p. 68).

Alongside those whose picture of health highlights a sense of belonging or connection, are others whose ideas capture the absurd, the sublime and the whimsical. There is the building that appears to be filled with jellyfish, once dusk falls, from multimedia artists Walter & Zoniel (p. 169). Photographer David Parker wonders about the man in his image of a shimmering blue car in a ditch in the Nazca desert in southern Peru (p. 154). Did the man tip his Chevy over the levee, or did it fall from outer space into a land where a lost civilisation has etched lines that have made folk wonder about aliens before? Animators Kyne Uhlig and Nikolaus Hillebrand sent a photograph of fresh vegetables waiting patiently at a bus stop in Germany. For the pair these life-sized veg make a statement about local transport and the climate-damaging impact of excessive food miles of an otherwise healthy diet (p. 112).

I have spent much of my professional life seeking answers to the classic six questions of journalism: *who? what? where? when? how?* and, most importantly for me, *why?* When seeking the *why?* of this collection, the answer is not straightforward. But if it raises your thoughts to see hope beyond the numbing horror of war and the residual anxieties of global pandemic, then perhaps that is answer enough. I hope you enjoy flicking through the pages of this book and perhaps find something that encourages you to ponder your own picture of health.

Susan Watts is an award-winning journalist who spent nearly two decades at the BBC's Newsnight programme covering science, technology, the environment and medicine, and their political and social impact. Susan is a former Head of Communications and Engagement at the LMS, a director of the Scottish Association for Marine Science in Oban, and a physics graduate of Imperial College London.

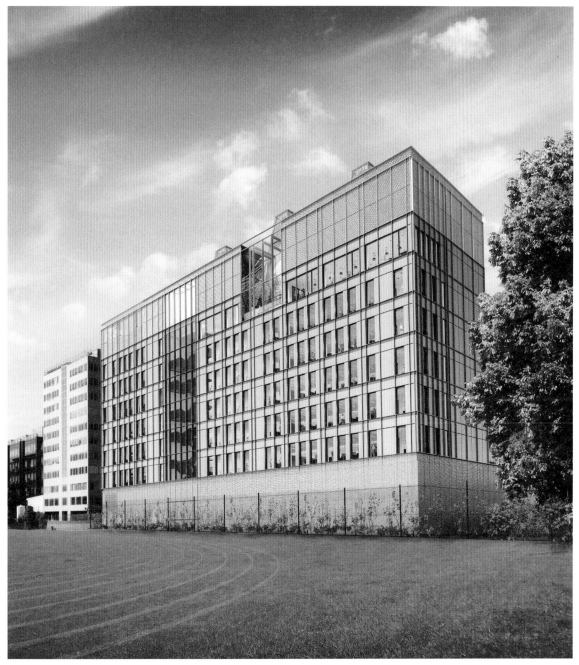

An artist's impression of the new building. Credit: Ark Visuals

Chris Beckley
TABLE TENNIS COACH

My total dedication is to support and help everyone to experience the amazing joys, participation, performance benefits, fun, laughter, creativity, friendship, community sense of belonging, team spirit, happiness, wellness (and much more) by playing the wonderful sport of table tennis – regardless of abilities, gender, race, or social or financial background. By providing low cost coaching sessions to both children and adults, a table tennis club offers loads of fun for members of all ages to learn bat, ball, and hand and eye co-ordination skills and, more importantly, raise their fitness levels, get active and stay healthy.

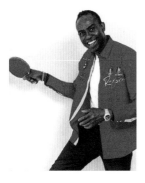

I've played table tennis since I can remember being a little boy...the passion was natural, and I was totally immersed even at a young age. I still managed to pursue and obtain a reasonably good education followed by a career in the training and development department of the London Fire Brigade that lasted a good and meritorious 26 years. Four years to date I'm a full time and totally lucky, happy and privileged licenced table tennis coach with so many clients and participants across two London boroughs – Hackney and Islington. And I have recently won the National Table Tennis Men's Volunteer of the Year Award.

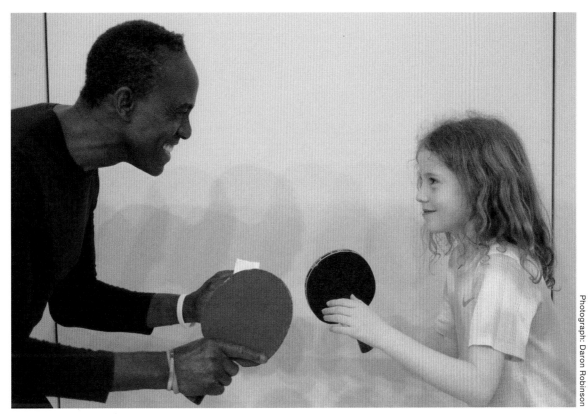

Ottoline Leyser

CHIEF EXECUTIVE UKRI

Health has many dimensions. This picture, of my niece with a kite, in the green outdoors, on a beautiful day, captures many of them. It is full of joie de vivre.

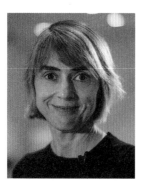

Professor Dame Ottoline Leyser is Chief Executive of UKRI and Regius Professor of Botany, University of Cambridge. Previously Director of the Sainsbury Laboratory, Cambridge, she has made important contributions to the understanding of plant hormones. She has also worked extensively in science policy, serving, for example as Chair of the Nuffield Council on Bioethics. She is a Fellow of the Royal Society, a Member of the Leopoldina and European Molecular Biology Organization, and an International Member of the US National Academy of Sciences. In 2017 she was appointed DBE for services to plant science, science in society and equality and diversity in science.

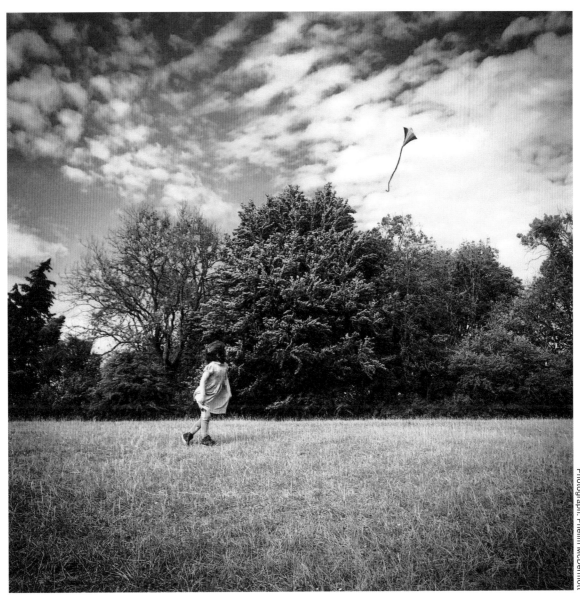

Sian Harding

CARDIAC PHARMACOLOGIST

This is an image of a cardiac muscle cell stained to show the muscle striation pattern: its length is around the thickness of a human hair. I've been fascinated by the cardiomyocyte for more than 30 years. The structure is so beautiful, and their ability to beat in the culture dish for hours is amazing.

Being able to study the individual cells gave us the ability to use many sophisticated imaging and molecular methods. Looking at the human cardiomyocyte from failing hearts provided a deep insight into the changes during heart failure and led to many discoveries.

Now, we are able to produce cardiomyocytes from human stem cells, but it has proved elusive to reproduce this intricate structure completely.

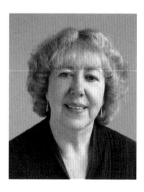

Sian Harding is Emeritus Professor of Cardiac Pharmacology at Imperial College London. She developed methods for isolating single cardiac muscle cells (cardiomyocytes) from human hearts and measuring their contractile function. She has been involved in gene and stem cell therapy for heart failure. Professor Harding also leads the Artworks Committee for Imperial College.

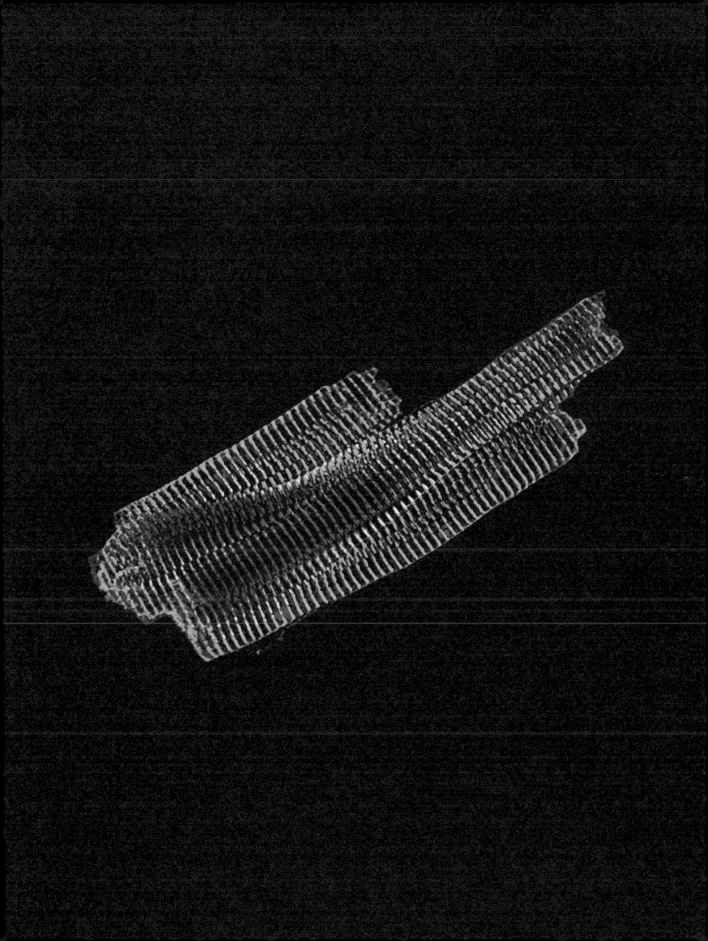

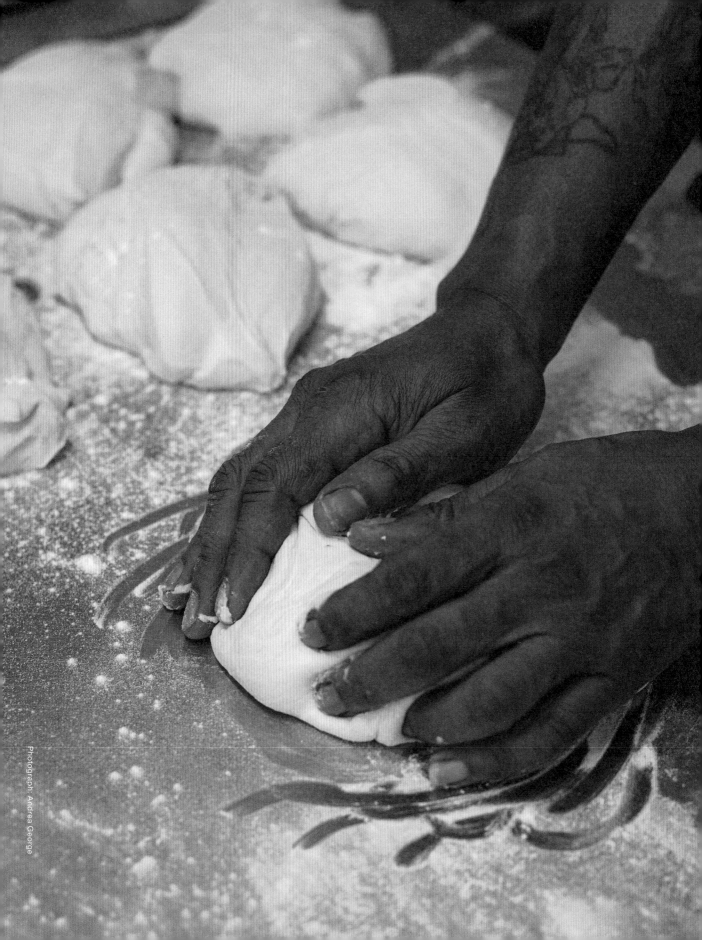

Robert Hunningher

BAKER

Bread is the epitome of health. The healthy grain, that grows and is harvested and milled to make the flour. The healthy sourdough starter, where wild yeast and good bacteria bubble and rise within the jar. A loaf successfully rising under the heat in the oven. Family and friends around a dinner table where bread has been a staple for over a millennium. Even today, people turned to making bread during the pandemic to help their mental health, distracted by the life blooming in their starter jars and the age-old craft – including me!

Life is a challenge and everyone on their path faces struggles, some more so than others. For some life is simply survival. It was our struggles through the pandemic that led me to bake my first loaf of sourdough and open our Humdingers bakery to help those not just struggling themselves but trying to survive. The sales of our sourdough bread fund our soup kitchen which we run four days a week to ensure families and children don't go to bed hungry, because what is healthy about that?

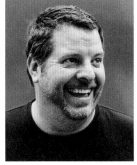

Having cut his teeth in the industry, working as a chef in some of London's finest restaurants, Robert Hunningher founded Humdingers Catering in 2009 with a vision to bring unpretentious but delicious food to as many people as possible. Based on Hoxton Street

in East London, the business consists of Humdingers Catering and Humdingers Bakery & Soup Kitchen. When the pandemic hit, it became an opportunity for Robert to give back to the local community and to date, the soup kitchen funded by the bakery has served

over 300,000 meals, earning him a British Empire Medal awarded by the Queen.

Steve Gschmeissner
ELECTRON MICROSCOPIST

Stem cells are the wonder cells of the human body. They are the raw materials, from which all other cells are generated, including those with specialised functions, such as blood, brain, muscle or bone cells. No other cell in the body has the natural ability to generate new cell types.

Their unique ability to regenerate and repair damaged tissue has led to one of the greatest medical breakthroughs of the modern era – stem cell therapy. This exciting area of biomedical research has the potential to provide treatments for some of the most intractable and devastating diseases such as cancer, diabetes and Alzheimer's.

This image is produced using a scanning electron microscope (SEM). It shows the precise moment the stem cell separates to form two daughter cells.

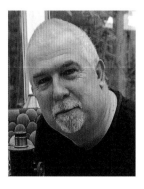

Internationally renowned electron microscopist Steve Gschmeissner has created an astonishing collection of high-power, false-coloured images of specimens ranging from diatoms to cancer cells to new materials. Published globally in all types of media, his work was most famously adapted by Damien Hirst in the artist's 'Biopsy series'. Combining a deep understanding of the science behind the specimen with a strong visual awareness, his breath-taking images have won numerous prestigious awards, including the 2021 Lennart Nilsson Award for extraordinary image makers in science.

Stem cells by Stephen Gschmeissner,
courtesy of Science Photo Library

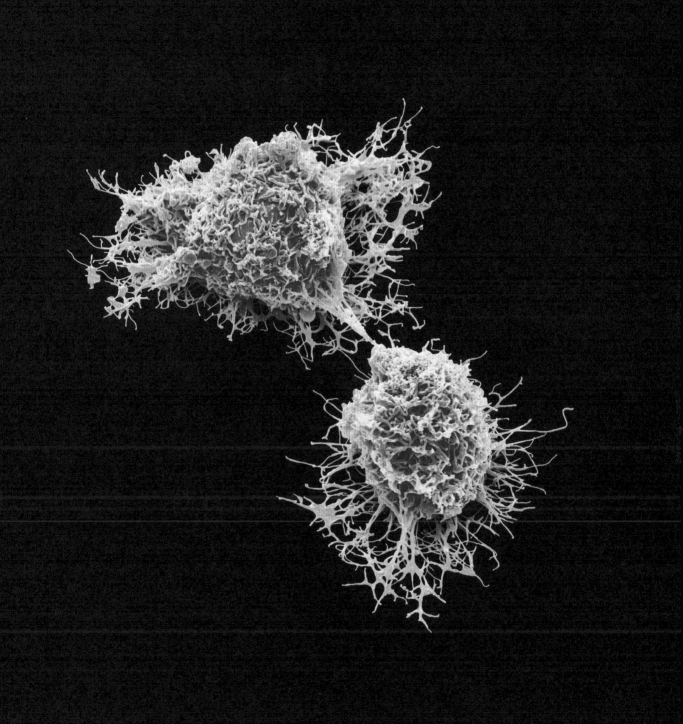

Heidi Williamson

POET

A microbiome is a community of micro-organisms – the human microbiome consists of bacteria, bacteriophage, fungi, protozoa and viruses that live in and on us. The ghazal ('guzzle') is an ancient Arabic verse form where each couplet ends on the same word or phrase, preceded by a rhyme. The last couplet includes a proper name.

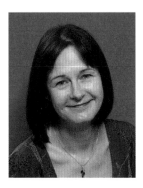

Heidi Williamson is an Advisory Fellow for the Royal Literary Fund, and teaches for the Poetry School, Poetry Society and others. She has been Poet-in-Residence at the London Science Museum's Dana Centre, the John Jarrold Printing Museum, and RLF Fellow at the University of East Anglia. She has three award-winning poetry collections with Bloodaxe Books.

Microbiome ghazal

Here too are dreaming landscapes...
Here too are the masses
tillers of the soil.
In the Microscope, MIROSLAV HOLUB

How little the average *us* knows about what goes on inside
our own bodies. We deny the existence of trillions of lives there – inside.

How rarely we think of their minuscule schemes. We seldom discuss them.
Meanwhile, every second, whole habitats of unseen species flare inside

our guts, eyebrows, skin... Our own intimate bacteria, protozoa, fungi, viruses
passed on to us like genes. If we could open up and stare inside

we'd see the chemical communities, currents, and settings that shape us.
If we witnessed what our partner, our friend, our enemy wears inside

we might see ensembles we have in common. A skin that attaches
only to itself is miserly. I imagine it peaceful, but perhaps it's warfare inside:

each strand bound by loyalty to its own kin, whatever that is. This messy vision
of shapes, this clutter of colours and actions, like some vast fairground inside,

makes my head spin. They could be our primal guides, if only we knew
how to listen. They go about their business, but I hear language is rare inside.

They're more copious than our cells – so who possesses who is a delicate question.
I suspect we're not gracious hosts, but I wonder if they care. Inside,

they protect themselves, and us. Without us, they're orphaned, or worse.
Without them, we can't mind our own body or care for its welfare inside.

This conglomerate called *Heidi*, what is it really? I'm not even CEO.
Still, my microbiome, this unsung company – it sustains me knowing they're inside.

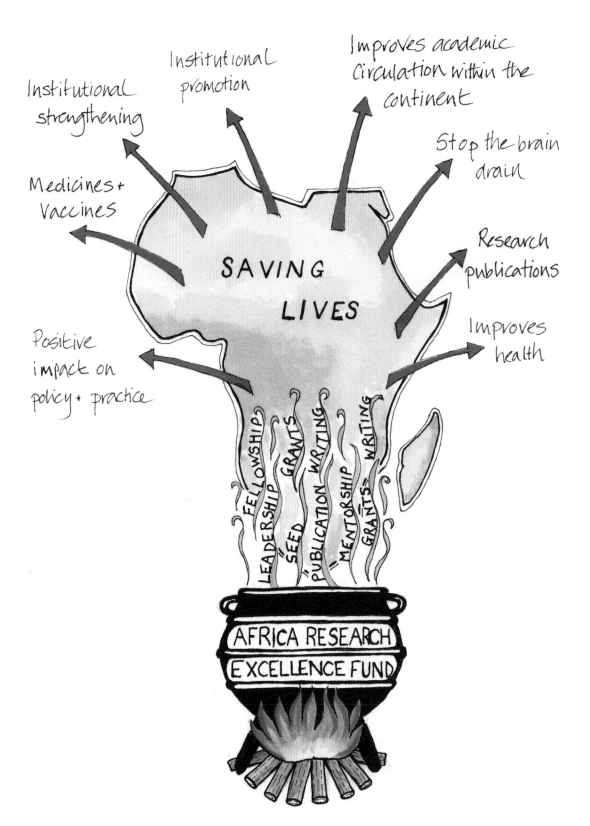

Africa – another hot spot for science research and discovery. Illustration: Nicky Beaumont

Tumani Corrah

GLOBAL HEALTH PRACTITIONER

For global health to become truly global, every corner of our world must bring relevant contributions to the table. Today, Africa's population of 1.25 billion whilst representing 17% of the world's population, shoulders 25% of the global disease burden and contributes only 3% of global scientific publications. The projected increase of the continent's population to 6 billion over the next 100 years, together with climate change, deforestation and increased air travel spells doom and gloom for the future of health and healthcare in Africa.

With the increasing numbers of research laboratories, the time is right to invest in talented emerging African scientists by providing them with stepping stones to become future scientific leaders who stay and carry out their science in the continent. To achieve this, Africa's talented emerging health researchers require the knowledge and skills to ask compelling research questions, the ability to design their own research, skills to collect their own data and samples and the competence to analyse and interpret these. Only in this way can they grow to become established independent health researchers with international recognition. This emerging African talent, working together with returning world renowned African scientists from the diaspora will form equitable partnerships with colleagues from the North to drive science from within Africa, science that will improve health and save lives GLOBALLY.

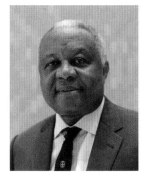

Professor Tumani Corrah KBE is Emeritus Director of the MRC Unit The Gambia at the London School of Hygiene & Tropical Medicine and Founder and President of the Africa Research Excellence Fund (AREF). Established just over five years ago, AREF focuses on talented emerging postdoctoral and clinician health researchers in the continent providing them with stepping stones to a successful research career in Africa for Africa. Research that will impact on policies to improve health and save lives in Africa and globally.

Angela Palmer
ARTIST

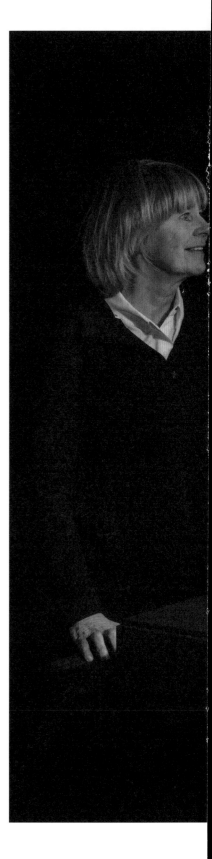

The sphere that changed the world is an ethereal rendering of the SARS-CoV-2 coronavirus: you are confronted by the entire sphere, with its protein spikes emerging from the surface, but as you pass around, it disappears entirely from view, only to reappear, echoing the elusive behaviour of the virus as it continues to spread around the world.

The installation may prompt reflection and contemplation of loss – a loss that will of course be unique to each of us. Laid bare, at eight million times its size, the particle may also offer empowerment and agency seen suspended and imprisoned in glass, open to scrutiny and interrogation. The deadly and elusive entity is suddenly rendered solitary, isolated and vulnerable, unsettlingly mirroring the condition it has imposed, and continues to impose, on us ourselves.

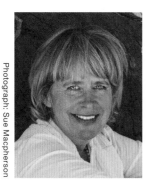

Photograph: Sue Macpherson

Angela Palmer is a sculptor with works in the permanent collections of museums worldwide, including The Smithsonian Air and Space Museum; The Science Museum, London; The Ashmolean; The National Galleries of Scotland; and the Wellcome Trust. Mapping is at the core of her work and using a technique she developed she draws or engraves details from cross-sections onto multiple sheets of glass which are then stacked to create a sculptural three-dimensional drawing in space. She recently recreated the original Wuhan coronavirus particle, eight million times its size, and separately one of its spikes, upscaled 11 million times.

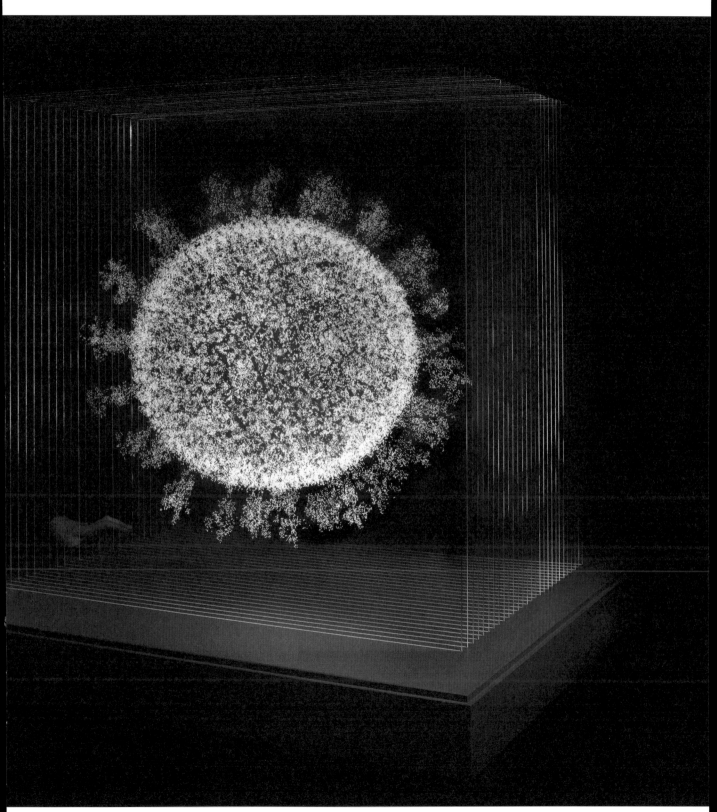

The SARS-CoV-2 virus, a 3D engraving on glass. Photograph: Andrew Smart of A.C.Cooper, London

Xiaomeng (Mona) Xu 徐晓梦
SOCIAL, HEALTH AND TEACHING PSYCHOLOGIST

This is a photo I took at Zion National Park, the first time I went backpacking. It was a challenging and intense time that has become a cherished memory. When I think of health, I'm reminded of all the great things about that trip. Being in nature, surrounded by beauty. Sharing a new adventure with wonderful friends. Taking a real break from work, screens, and urgency. Resting. Living in the moment. Pushing outside comfort zones, learning, and revelling in being alive. May all our futures be filled with these experiences.

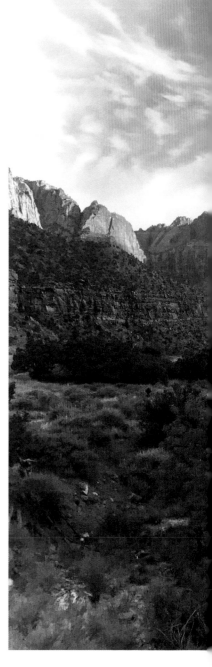

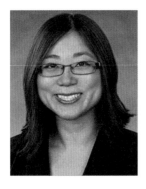

Xiaomeng is an Associate Professor in Experimental Psychology at Idaho State University. Xiaomeng combines health, social and neuropsychology research to explore the factors that influence our behavioural health and close romantic relationships.

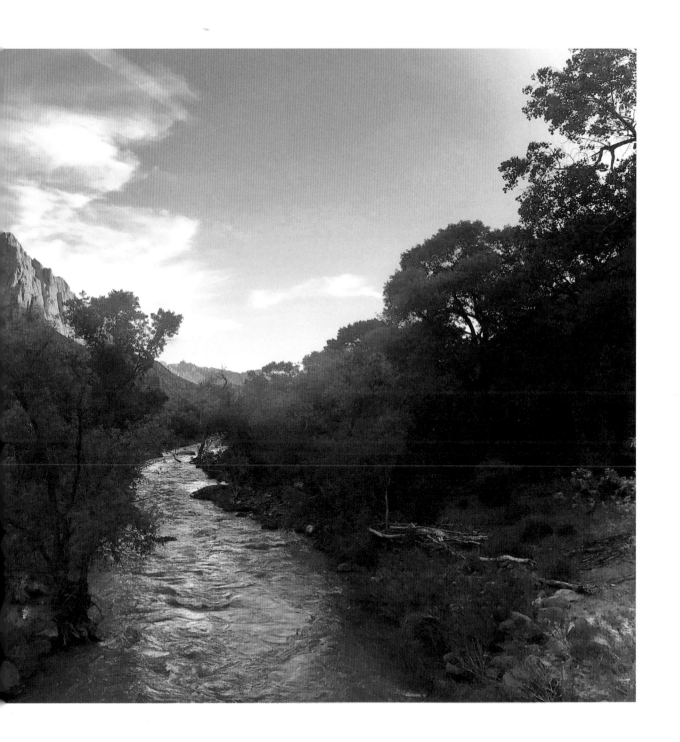

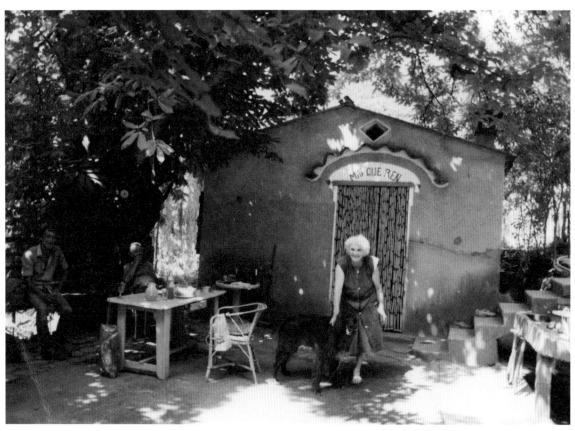

Above the door it says, 'better than nothing'. Photographs: Janet Mata

David Stubbs

ECOLOGIST

In the early 1980's I was living in a small village in the foothills of the Massif des Maures in southern France, doing an ecological study of wild tortoises. During a pause in my fieldwork, I enjoyed dropping in on Victor and Lucienne Rosso at their summer 'cabanon'. It was an enchanting place tucked away up a short track.

Theirs was a simple life, but one that was full of contentment and acceptance of the natural world around them. They were among the last of a generation that had known the traditional ways of Provençal life and how to work the land, cultivate and harvest in balance with nature. For me they were a window into a past way of life that spoke of an ecological richness and heritage that was rapidly disappearing. Chatting with them by their cabanon I appreciated their generosity of spirit and understanding of the world around them, which for me embodied a picture of health.

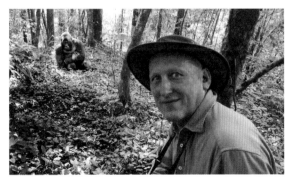

David exploring in Uganda

David Stubbs has had a life-long passion for the natural world. He trained as an ecologist, but his career evolved from pure conservation biology towards more applied environmental management topics, especially in the sport sector. He became the Head of Sustainability for the London 2012 Olympic and Paralympic Games and is now a leading global sustainability expert in the sport and event sectors. He lives in a small village in rural Norfolk, UK, with his wife Jan, two dogs and several pairs of swifts nesting in his roof.

Dulcie Rodrigues

MRI DEPARTMENT ADMINISTRATOR

I chose these two pictures to illustrate what to me a picture of health is (or should be) and therefore conducive to healthy living. The first is a picture of myself at a friend's wedding. A happy, fun and stress-free occasion. My view is that if you try to live a stress-free life and look at life's positives rather than negatives, then life, for me and you, will be a picture of health.

The second picture I have chosen is a pitcher filled with healthy goodness. We are told that if we do not abuse our bodies but imbibe of nature's goodness, we can all live happy and healthy lives. Good advice – if we take it!!

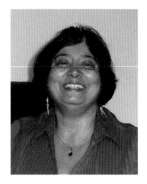

I joined the magnetic resonance imaging facility in June 1987 initially on a nine-month contract and I'm still here 35 years later. I arrived in London on a cold and damp January afternoon in 1984 from warm and sunny Pakistan to begin a new life – and what a life it has been. In this research environment I have met and worked with the most wonderful people and have been educated a lot as a result of my association with them. The highlight of my life now is being a grandmother to my 6-year-old granddaughter.

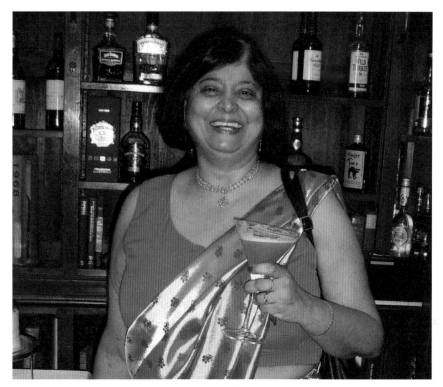

A picture of health

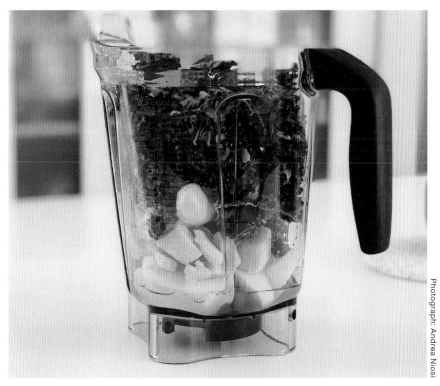

A pitcher of health

Photograph: Andrea Niosi

31

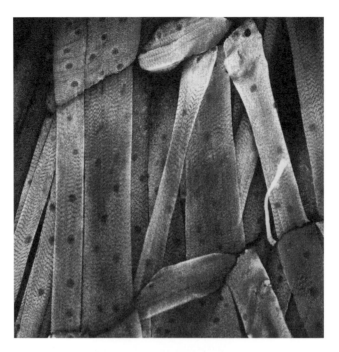

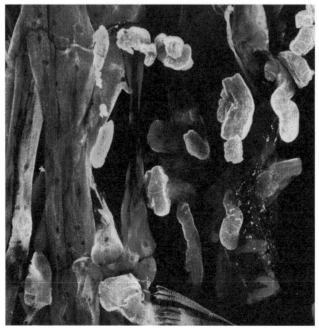

Susumu Hirabayashi

BIOLOGIST

Healthy muscles let you do things you enjoy doing: walking, running, cooking, playing sports and playing musical instruments.

Skeletal muscle is the largest organ in our body. It is a highly adaptable tissue that can enlarge its mass in response to exercise and nutrition. Conversely, a progressive loss of skeletal muscle mass and function can occur in chronic diseases such as obesity and cancer (cachexia), or ageing (sarcopenia). These muscle wasting diseases are associated with increased mortality and diminished quality of life. With the global increase in ageing population, obesity, and cancer, muscle wasting disease is a rapidly growing clinical issue.

Research using *Drosophila* (fruit flies) has found that diets high in sugar not only lead to obesity and promote cancer progression, but also promote muscle weakness (lower image, highlighting two proteins in muscle cells in red and green). Our research is aimed at understanding how a healthy diet can maintain healthy muscles (upper image) and prevent the muscles from wasting.

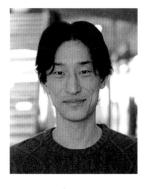

Susumu Hirabayashi completed a PhD at the Tokyo Medical and Dental University (Tokyo, Japan), followed by a three-year appointment as a research staff scientist. For his postdoc, he moved to Mount Sinai School of Medicine (New York, USA), where he studied the link between obesity and cancer, using Drosophila as a model system. In 2014, he established his own research group (Metabolism and Cell Growth group) at the LMS, to investigate host-tumour metabolic and nutritional interactions.

Mimi White

ROCK CLIMBER

Climbing has become such a big part of my life that I now could not function without it. It connects me to the outdoors and has become the thing that drives and motivates me in everything I do. I have been climbing for nearly four years now: it has shaped my future in ways I couldn't have imagined, and the climbing community has been such a huge part of my journey.

Rock climbing: The pursuit of an essentially pointless yet incredibly simple task has several aspects that I get so much from. Encouraging me to spend huge amounts of time outdoors in beautiful places has done wonders for my mental health.

Exercising through problem-solving, "How do I get up this piece of rock?" with only the available surfaces and my physical ability has helped me completely change my objectives for exercise and health. I no longer want to train to change my shape, motivated by insecurity and popular preferences in pursuit of a 'beach body' or 'hourglass figure'. I'm driven to train to enhance my physical ability and optimise my health because the challenge and intrinsic motivation are so rewarding. In my journey with climbing, I went from a fragile runner who had a problematic relationship with food to a driven, muscular, stronger individual with much clearer and healthier goals.

I get so much enjoyment from climbing and it makes me feel so strong, capable and powerful.

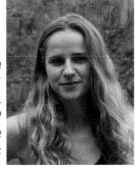

Photograph: Tom Stockton

Mimi is currently at Bangor University training to be a Sports Psychologist qualified to help others with their mental health, and to coach climbing, while continuing her own journey with climbing.

Night Climbing. Photograph: Marc Langley

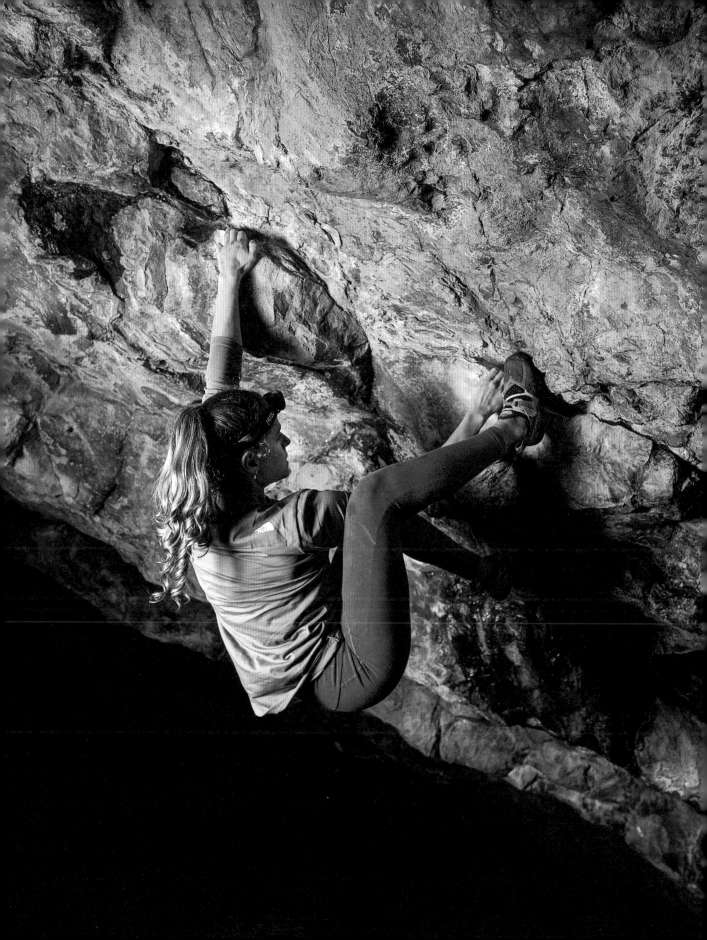

**High-Intensity
Interval Training
Open Goal**

11:05 - 11:52

Total Time

0:46:56

Active Kilocalories

343KCAL

Total Kilocalories

429KCAL

Avg Heart Rate

150BPM

Heart Rate

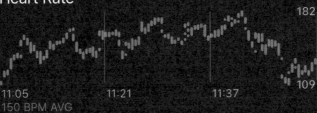

182

109

11:05   11:21   11:37

150 BPM AVG

Sue Black

COMPUTER SCIENTIST

I love technology and how it connects us to each other and in this case to my own health. Just as having access to my banking data through a mobile app gives me better awareness of my financial situation, having access to my fitness data gives me better awareness of my health and how to improve it.

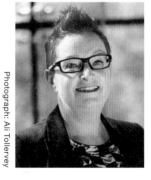

Sue Black OBE is Professor of Computer Science and Technology Evangelist at Durham University, a government advisor and Trustee at Comic Relief. She set up the first on-line network for women in tech, BCSWomen, and led the campaign to save Bletchley Park. She has championed women in tech for over two decades, founding #techmums and the pioneering TechUPWomen retraining women into tech careers. Having left school at 16 and married at 20, Sue went to university as a single parent of three children at 27, gaining a degree in computing then a PhD in software engineering.

Ian Needleman

PERIODONTIST

Oral health has profound impacts on the way people lead their lives. Our mouths are our shop windows, strongly linked with our confidence and self-esteem. Oral health affects physical health and vice versa. This is most strongly demonstrated by the negative effects that diabetes can have on oral health and in the opposite direction, poor oral health can impair blood sugar control. As you might expect, the burden of poor oral health is greatest in disadvantaged communities with disproportionate effects on life quality and general health.

Having studied the effects of oral health, and with a personal love of sport, we were interested to explore the oral health of those remarkable gods and goddesses also known as elite athletes, and its relationship with performance. After large studies at London 2012, Premier League Football and Olympic and professional athletes prior to Rio 2016, we found a consistent and troubling message. Oral diseases (tooth decay, gum diseases and tooth erosion) were common and around a third of athletes reported negative effects from this on performance. We are currently looking into the mechanisms of these impairments. Alongside the psychological effects of poor oral health, we are finding effects on respiratory and possibly cognitive function. We are also interested in the inflammation that oral diseases cause elsewhere in the body. Fortunately, we have also shown that these impacts can be improved by simple changes that athletes (and anyone else) can make.

Treasure oral health to reduce inequalities and promote a better life.

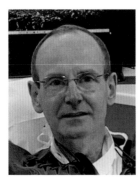

Ian is Professor of Periodontology and Evidence-Informed Healthcare at University College London. He leads the Centre for Oral Health and Performance, which was awarded recognition by the International Olympic Committee as part of the UK Research Centre for Prevention of Injury and Protection of Athlete Health. He is also in specialist practice and a Cochrane Editor for Periodontal Health. He has been awarded many prizes for his research, teaching and leadership. During the pandemic he helped develop a Family Liaison Team service for University College London Hospital Critical Care Unit. He is a keen road and mountain runner when not injured.

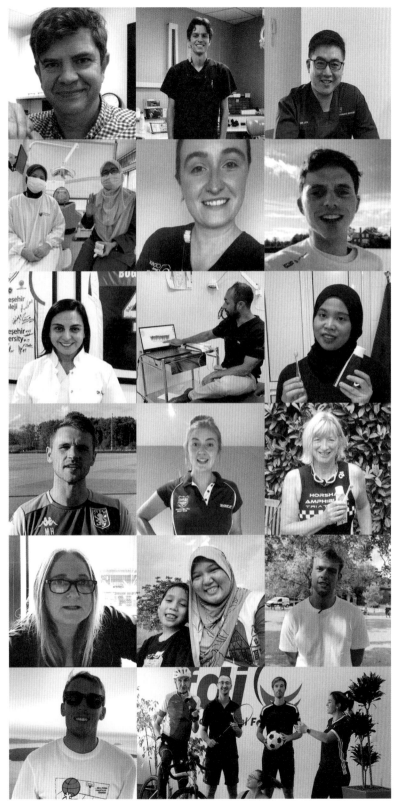

Dentists and athletes passionate about oral health and performance

Wilf Walker
MUSIC PROMOTER

This is a photograph of my grandmother, Celestine, with seven of her eight great-grandchildren. She was 92 when this picture was taken and she lived for another seven years, missing out on turning 100 by five months. If ever there was a literal picture of health it is this photo of a smiling, happy and healthy family.

Celestine was a strong and lively woman. She was born in Antigua in 1903 on the same plantation where her mother was born and despite being hard of hearing and diabetic her whole life, she was always enterprising and hard working. In our village in Trinidad she raised chickens and sold the eggs, made ice-cream on Sundays and sold it to kids and she took in washing for an English family. As a boy I would deliver and collect this washing balanced in a tray on my head every Saturday. She also ran an enterprise where a group of women all paid in some money each week, with all the contributions being handed out to one person in the group a month. She did all this at the same time as looking after myself and my three sisters and brother.

She was the hub of her community and was the most caring person in my life as a child growing up in Trinidad. This caring nature was enjoyed by her great-grandchildren who greatly benefitted from having Celestine in their lives. We've all got her strong genes in our family. Her only child, my mother, is 95 years old and still alive today. I look forward to seeing a similar picture of myself with my great-grandchildren in many years' time – Celestine is a picture and an inspiration of health!

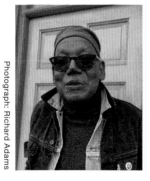

Photograph: Richard Adams

Born in Trinidad, in 1945 Wilf moved to West London aged 16. With no school qualifications, a 3-year prison sentence and severe mental health breakdowns in his mid-twenties behind him he went on to inspire others and make huge contributions to developing live black music in the UK and internationally. For over 30 years, he produced live shows and tours for some of the world's most respected live acts. His many achievements include initiating the live music stages at the Notting Hill Carnival (1979–1993) and organising the first Free Nelson Mandela benefit concert. In 2012 he received an OBE for forty years of promoting live black music.

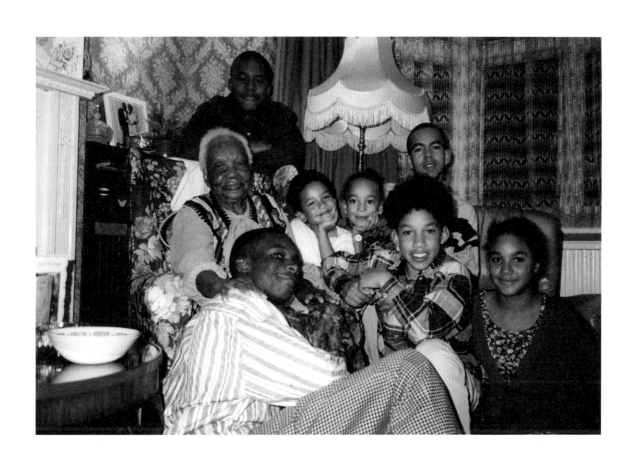

Mervyn King
ECONOMIST

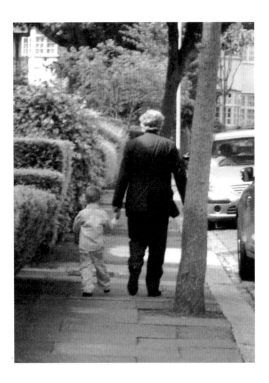

The older generation supporting the younger?
The younger generation supporting the older?
The older and younger generations walking through life together.

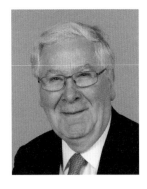

Governor of the Bank of England (2003–2013), Mervyn King studied at King's College Cambridge, taught at Cambridge and Birmingham Universities, and from 1984 was Professor of Economics at the London School of Economics. Currently he is the Alan Greenspan Professor of Economics and Professor of Law at New York University. Knighted in 2011, made a life peer in 2013, and in 2014 appointed as Knight of the Garter, he has published several books including The End of Alchemy, *and recently with John Kay,* Radical Uncertainty. *He is Chair of the Philharmonia Orchestra.*

Michael Rosen

POET

I watch myself from the ceiling
of a hospital ward.
I am still.
Inert.
Tubes running into my arm
into my nose and my throat.
I am being made better.

It's night.
A nurse takes my blood pressure
then my oxygen saturation.
She observes me.
Reads some figures
lit up on a screen.
She writes them down.
I am being made better.

Now my place on the ceiling
to watch myself
is at a rehab hospital:
I hold a frame.
Three people are there
to coach me
or catch me.
I take a step.
It's the first step.
I am being made better.

Michael Rosen is one of Britain's best loved writers and performance poets. He was the Children's Laureate from 2007-2009 and has published over 200 books for children and adults. As a presenter for radio and television and as a political columnist, his main theme is education, the writing and performance almost always spiked with humour. He is currently Professor of Children's Literature at Goldsmiths, University of London.

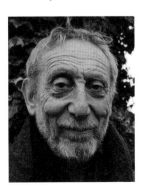

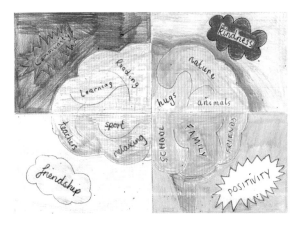

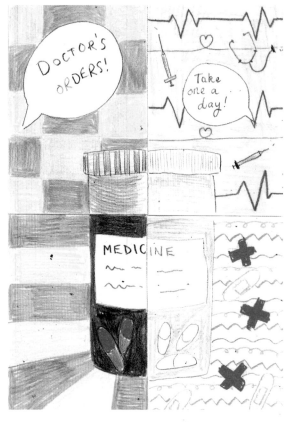

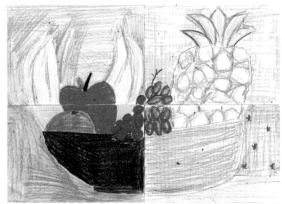

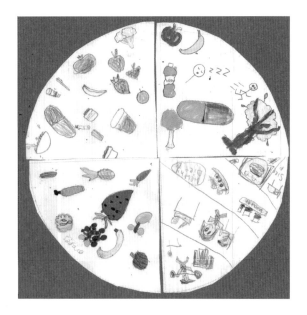

Think About . . .

Think about health,
Not wealth
Think about yourself and others
Think about your family,
Sister and brothers

Put yourself in others' shoes
Remember all the don'ts and do's
Push yourself to be phenomenal
And eventually you'll be unstoppable

We should be happy and free,
And that's what we should truly be
Never forget to always be kind
And surely friends you will find

Think about you . . .
And be true!

Old Oak Primary School

Scientists from the LMS visited our school to deliver a series of workshops in which students got to explore cells and learn about cutting edge research that seeks to improve human health. This helped spark the students' ideas of what *A Picture of Health* is to them and here we present their interpretations of the phrase.

The poem *Think About...* was written by some Year 6 (aged 10–11) pupils who took ideas from children in Early Years and Key Stage 1. It is grounded in family, behaviour and emotion and demonstrates the maturity of these young children's world view. The circle was made by some children in Year 3 and depicts fruit, sleep, exercise and tooth-brushing – all the things we encourage children to think about at this age when it comes to keeping healthy! The three mosaic images were done by children in Year 4 and 5. They depict a bowl of fruit, a brain annotated with the things they feel contribute to their overall health, and a medicine bottle with striking graphic patterns.

Old Oak Primary School is based in East Acton, just a stone's throw away from the LMS. We are a school grounded in progress and community. We believe our school is a special place where we are committed to providing the best for each and every child here, creating a friendly and inclusive atmosphere. Educating the 'whole child' remains a cornerstone of our values and our involvement in activities like this reflect that.

Jean-Baptiste Vannier

MOLECULAR BIOLOGIST

In each of our cells our unique genetic code exists as lengths of DNA sequence assembled as discrete structures called chromosomes. Chromosomes (here stained blue) end in DNA/protein structures called telomeres (red), repetitive sequences that protect genes along the chromosome from degradation.

Telomeres can become shorter with ageing, damage through stress and in disease, but they are also restorable. In 2009, Elizabeth Blackburn, Carol Greider and Jack Szostak shared the Nobel Prize in Physiology or Medicine for their discovery of telomerase, the enzyme that replenishes shortened telomeres by adding DNA sequence. Telomerase is not active in most of our body's cells, but in cancer cells the enzyme is usually reactivated conferring unlimited cell division. Cancer cells have developed mechanisms by which telomeres are constantly elongated, which is a key process in helping cancer cells to continue growing.

Keeping telomeres at their best is a critical feature of healthy ageing. Maintaining the balance between senescence/cell death and tumour formation is bound up with the mechanisms that control telomere shortening and lengthening. Hence, targeting telomere maintenance pathways in cancer is a long-term goal in my field, as we strive to keep humans healthier longer.

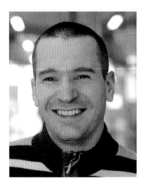

Dr Jean-Baptiste Vannier's interest is in the fundamental roles of the chromosome ends called telomeres. He established the Telomere Replication & Stability group at the LMS in 2014 and, as of 2021, now leads his group as an Imperial College Lecturer at the Institute of Clinical Sciences. As a well-recognised principal scientist in the telomere field with many fruitful collaborations with Imperial colleagues, he is concerned with the complex secondary structure adopted by telomere DNA as it is a potential source of genome instability, the hallmark of many diseases including cancer.

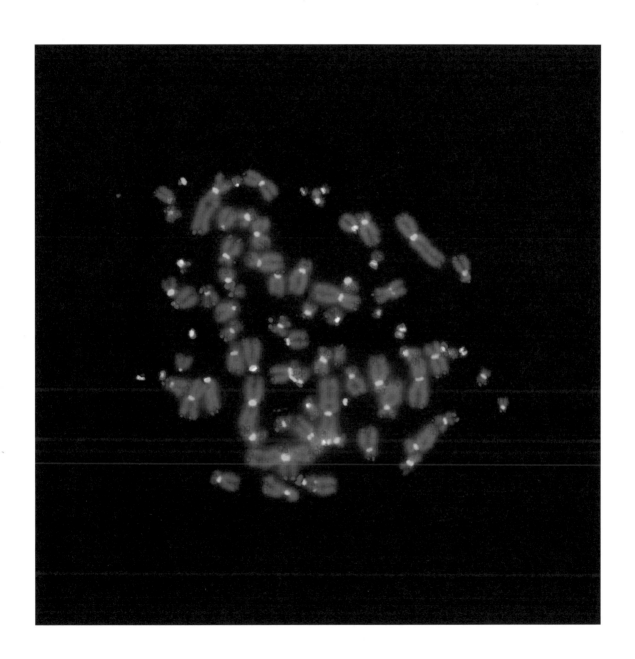

Asna Afghan
JUNIOR DOCTOR

This is a candid photo I took of my 65-year-old father during the peak of the COVID-19 pandemic. He would go on daily walks to keep himself fit and healthy in our local park. In this photo I have captured him reminiscing about his time as a professional javelin thrower. He is a type 2 diabetic and feels that his health has deteriorated significantly since his diagnosis. He had lost a lot of weight during this time and that is what he sees reflected in this image. However, in my opinion, this image demonstrates the strength and athleticism he has managed to retain to this day. Two different perceptions of health captured in one image.

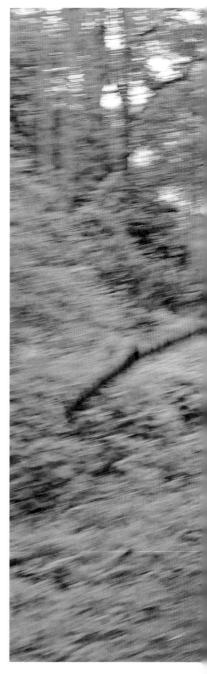

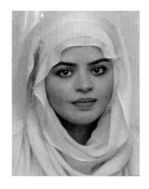

Newly qualified from Imperial College London, I am currently working in Renal Medicine at West London Renal and Transplant Centre, Hammersmith Hospital. It has always been my dream from a very young age to be a GP and this is still my dream today! I spend my free time engaging in various creative pursuits including photography, painting, Arabic calligraphy, graphic design, and photo editing. Throughout my life I have been heavily inspired by the honest, loving, and hardworking nature of my parents. Despite coming from nothing they have managed to raise four NHS doctors; an incredible achievement for which they deserve every recognition.

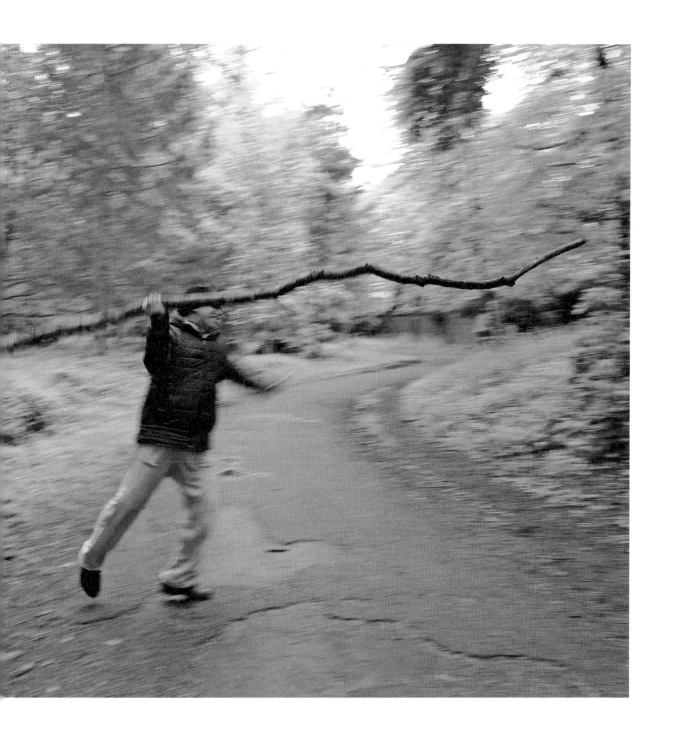

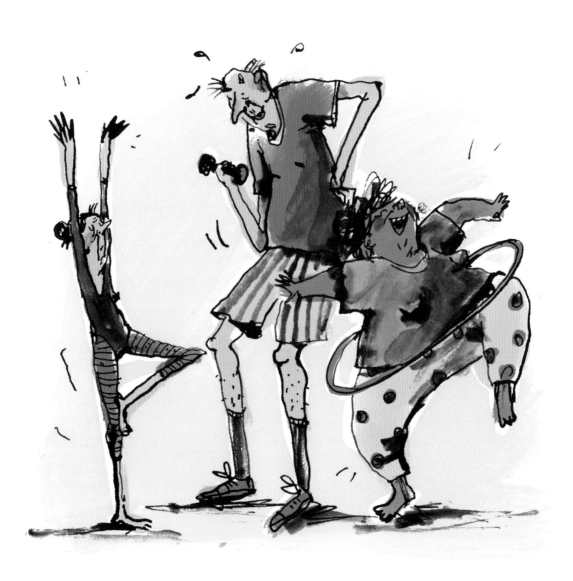

Elina Ellis

AUTHOR AND ILLUSTRATOR

People are usually scared of getting old. We associate old age with loneliness, decline and deterioration. I think this is the greatest misconception and we are missing the point. There is no 'use by' date on human beings! Yes, we grow older, but the emphasis should be on the word 'grow' and not on the word 'older', because we also grow wiser, kinder, more tolerant and more appreciative of life. We mature, evolve, expand and transform. My picture of health is the joy of living, the desire to grow and to contribute to the world not just till a certain age, but as long as we breathe.

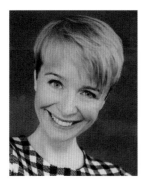

Elina Ellis is an award-winning picture books author and illustrator. Her books are published by top British, American and Canadian publishers and are translated into many languages and sold all over the world.

Isabel Oliver

CHIEF SCIENTIFIC ADVISOR TRANSITION LEAD

This is 'Smallpox Hill' close to where I live in Gloucestershire and not far from the home of Edward Jenner, the father of vaccines. It stands proudly separated from the Cotswold escarpment by a small valley which forms part of my early morning running route. Its proper name, which no one uses, is Downham Hill and it was the location of one of the earliest smallpox isolation hospitals. Local legend says that it played a role in Jenner's pioneering immunisation work. Who knows? What we know for a fact is that thanks to vaccination, smallpox, one of the most devastating diseases known to us was eliminated and that, since then, vaccines have saved millions of lives and given us much needed hope during the COVID-19 pandemic. In this difficult time, my daily runs and walks by Smallpox Hill have been key to my own wellbeing and the view of the beautiful avenue of sycamore trees in place of the isolation hospital on top of the hill a constant reminder of the wonderful health improvements that we have secured through vaccination and other scientific advancements.

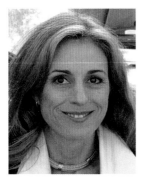

Professor Isabel Oliver was appointed Director of the National Infection Service in April 2020 having previously held other roles in Public Health England (PHE). She is also co-director of the National Institute for Health Research Health Protection Research Unit on Behavioural Science and Evaluation at the University of Bristol and Senior Medical Advisor to the COVID-19 NHS Test and Trace Programme. Having worked in acute hospital medicine, she completed public health specialist training becoming Regional Director of the Health Protection Agency in the South West before moving to PHE in 2013.

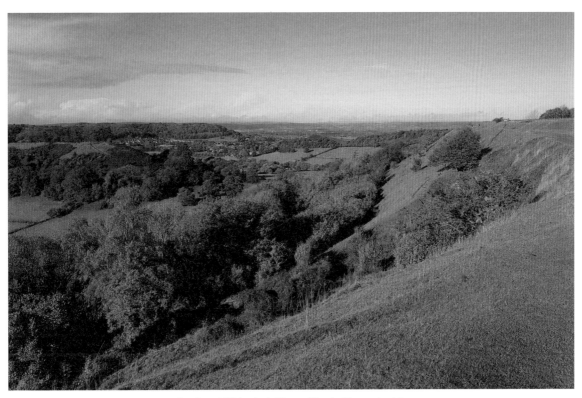

'Smallpox Hill' (to the left) near Uley in Gloucestershire

John Iredale

MRC INTERIM EXECUTIVE CHAIR

This is where I feel most at peace and most healthy. As a fragment of the ever threatened and shrinking true wilderness areas in the UK, it also feels like a place where nature and the planet is healthy.

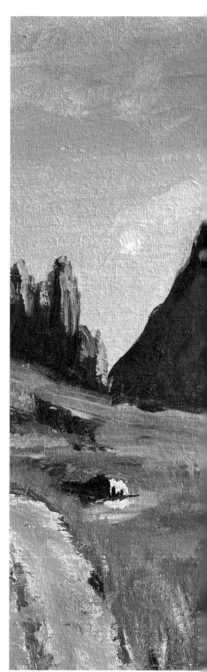

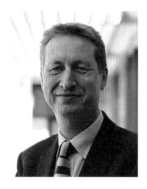

John Iredale graduated from the University of Southampton in 1985. He has since forged a career in academic medicine. A fellow of a number of academies and colleges including the Royal College of Physicians of both London and Edinburgh, he was previously

Regius Professor of Medical Science and Director of the Centre for Inflammation Research at the University of Edinburgh. He became a member of the MRC in 2016, before being asked to take the role of interim Executive Chair in 2022. He is a non-executive director

of the North Bristol NHS Trust, Professor of Medical Sciences at the University of Bristol, and a trustee of the British Heart Foundation.

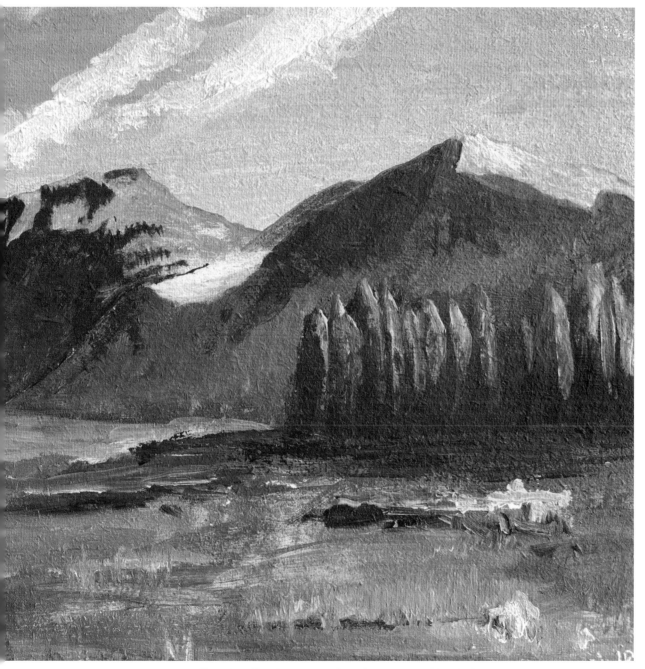

The trail to Fionn Loch, Wester Ross. Acrylic on board by John Iredale

Anne Howeson

ARTIST

These drawings mix fragments of my life with ideas about women's health across the centuries. The partially erased and redrawn earlier images – discovered in the print and photographic archives of the Wellcome Trust, London – were transformed into new narratives in response to the earlier material. The drawings were originally commissioned for the Wellcome Trust 'Stories' series 'Painful Realities,' which looked at endometriosis and pain.

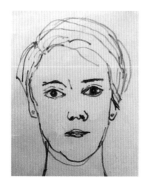

Jerwood Drawing Prize winner Anne Howeson has works in the collection of the Museum of London, The Guardian News and Media, St. George's Hospital and Imperial College. As a tutor at the Royal College of Art she promotes drawing as process outcome and a way of thinking.

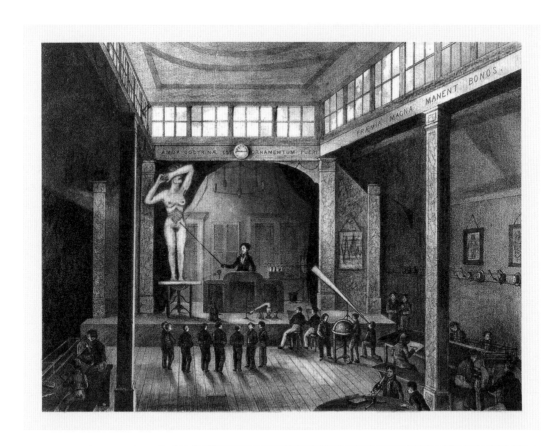

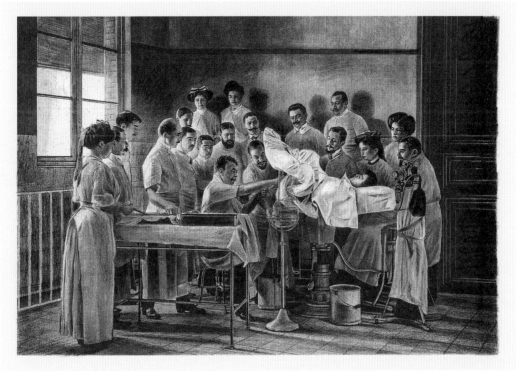

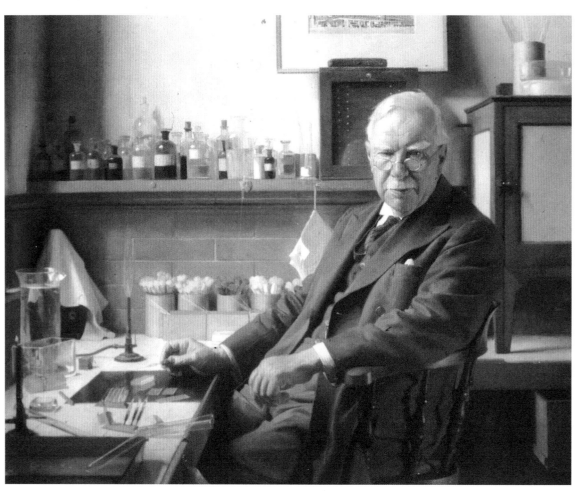

Portrait of Sir Almroth Wright by Gerald Kelly, 1934. Courtesy of the Alexander Fleming Laboratory Museum, Imperial College Healthcare NHS Trust

Jonathan Weber

INFECTIOUS DISEASES SPECIALIST

I have walked past this penetrating portrait of Almroth Wright almost every day for 30 years. To me, Wright represents world-leading scientific excellence, skill in training and practical innovation in microbiology – an area critical to global health and my own career in infectious diseases at St Mary's Hospital.

Born in 1861, Wright trained at Trinity College Dublin, moving to St Mary's Hospital in 1902 to establish a bacteriology research laboratory. His towering achievement was to develop the first inactivated vaccine for *Salmonella typhi*, test it on British troops serving in the second Boer war, then producing 10 million doses and persuading universal vaccination of all British troops in WW1. This population-level intervention was a pivotal moment in modern vaccinology.

Among Wright's trainees at St Mary's were Alexander Fleming (discovery of penicillin, 1928) and Leonard Colebrook (first successful treatment of puerperal fever – *Streptococcus pyogenes* – with sulphanilamide, 1935). Wright went on to focus on immunotherapy and was the first to publish on the risk of development of bacterial resistance to antibiotics; he died in 1947.

A noted misogynist and very public opponent of women's suffrage, Wright's reputation has been the subject of recent negative revision. My preferred position is not to write Wright out of history and memory, but rather to repudiate his misogyny by appointing women academics in his name.

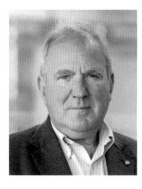

Dean, Faculty of Medicine at Imperial College London Professor Jonathan Weber trained at Cambridge University and Barts and took his PhD at the Institute of Cancer Research. He established the Genitourinary Medicine department at Imperial College in 1991. Since 1982 he has been researching HIV infection and AIDS and contributed to the development of antiretroviral therapy in the 1990's. Now he works on HIV prevention, including an HIV vaccine efficacy trial combining novel vaccines with pre-exposure prophylaxis. He is also Director of Imperial College Academic Health Science Centre which encompasses the seven major West London hospitals with the Institute of Cancer Research and Imperial College.

Jens Nielsen
SYSTEMS BIOLOGIST

Antibiotics have cured infections for decades and saved millions of lives since they were first discovered and used. But inevitably evolution finds a way of circumventing our existing drugs. Filamentous fungi produce natural products that have been exploited as pharmaceuticals. Penicillin was originally identified as a product of filamentous fungi and there are suspicions that these exquisite micro-organisms, may be a rich source of other important pharmaceuticals.

To identify the potential of filamentous fungi to produce products that can be screened for bioactivity, we performed whole genome-sequencing of 9 *Penicillium* species. By combining this new information with data on 15 published *Penicillium* genomes we identified 1,317 putative biosynthetic gene clusters (BGCs). Many of these BGCs contain genes encoding for either polyketides (PKS) or non-ribosomal peptide synthases (NRPS), which represent two classes of important enzymes engaged in production of a range of complex natural products. Penicillin, for example is produced by a NRPS, and the cholesterol lowering agent lovastatin is produced by a PKS. Our analysis identified more than 10 NRPS and 15 PKS in 24 species of *Penicillium*, showing that filamentous fungi have the capability to produce many more natural products than what has yet been discovered.

Celebrating the expanding horizon of fungal-derived pharmaceuticals, the new LMS cafe and roof terrace is festooned with this image from my lab – 'Fungal Salvation' on the LMS's BPoD described by Ruth Williams – reminding us to restock our antibiotic armoury.

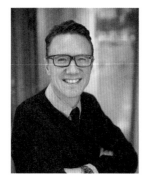

Jens Nielsen has a PhD (1989) from the Technical University of Denmark and joined Chalmers University of Technology, Sweden in 2008. He has been CEO of the BioInnovation Institute, Denmark since 2019. Inventor of 50+ patents and founder of several biotech companies, his work has produced natural rare molecules, antibiotics and biofuels. Recipient of numerous awards, including the Nature Mentoring Award, and the Eric and Sheila Samson Prime Minister's Prize for Innovation in Transportation Fuels, he is a member of several academies including the National Academy of Sciences in the USA, Royal Danish Academy of Science and Letters, and Chinese Academy of Engineering.

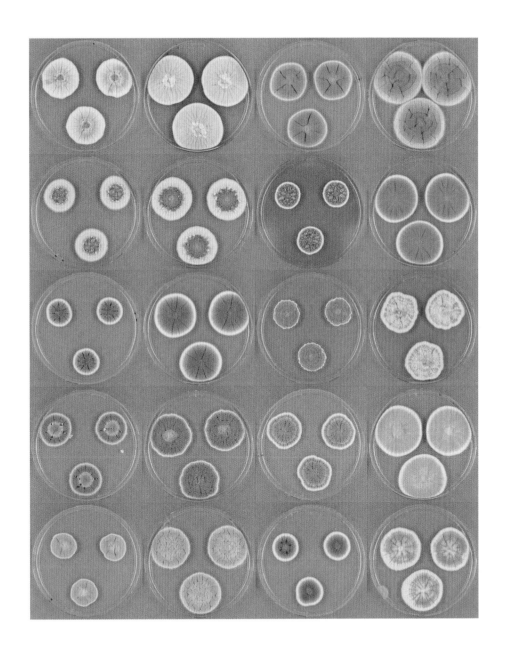

Helena Cochemé

BIOMEDICAL RESEARCHER

Metabolism is at the heart of life. With its vibrant brushstrokes, this picture captures in my mind the dynamic nature of metabolism. The combination of contrasting colours, from cool whites and blues to warm oranges and reds, evokes the flow of energy within living systems and the heat generated during biochemical reactions. This artwork has personal connections to the lab – it's an oil painting by Manfred Lennicke, father of post-doctoral researcher Dr Claudia Lennicke, and was recently featured on the cover of the scientific journal *Molecular Cell* accompanying a review article that we wrote together.

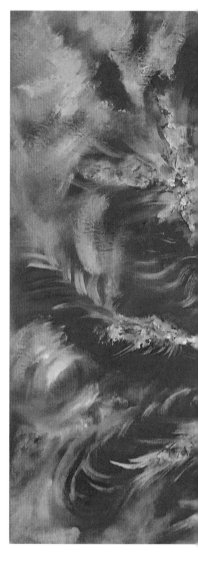

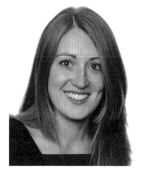

Dr Helena Cochemé is head of the Redox Metabolism group, established in 2013 at the LMS. She is also an Honorary Senior Lecturer at Imperial College London. Previously, she received her PhD in Biochemistry from the University of Cambridge in 2006, at the MRC Mitochondrial Biology Unit, followed by a post-doctoral position at the University College London Institute of Healthy Ageing from 2007. She uses the fruit fly Drosophila as a model to study ageing, with a particular focus on redox signalling and diet-induced metabolic diseases.

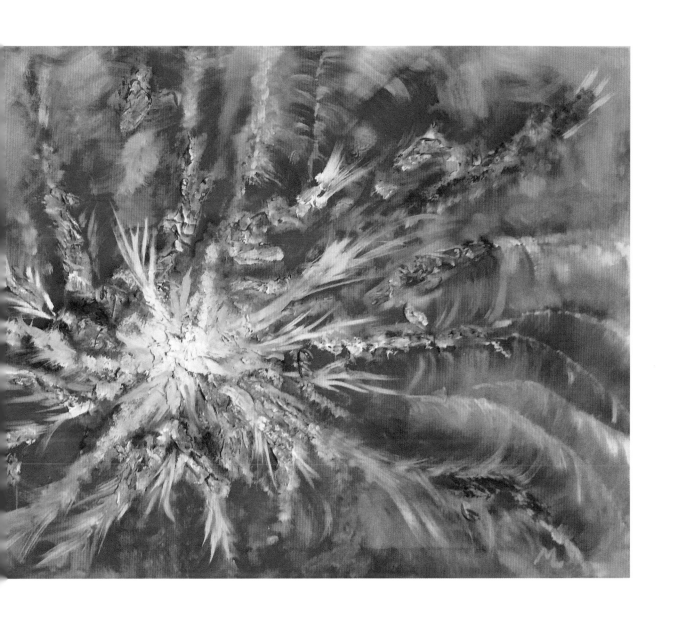

Sally Davies

PUBLIC AND GLOBAL HEALTH PRACTITIONER

Before Alexander Fleming discovered penicillin in 1928, an infection from a simple cut could mean the end of life. Thanks to antibiotics, we can treat previously life-threatening illnesses, such as pneumonia, meningitis and TB. Antibiotics form the backbone of our modern medicine, enabling safe cancer care, transplants and hip operations. But over time, bugs develop ways to escape the antibiotics that scientists have developed, rendering them ineffective. To save modern medicine and tackle this silent pandemic of Antimicrobial Resistance, we need to handle our precious antibiotics with care, using them sustainably and appropriately. We must also develop new treatments that target the most dangerous of infections. Without urgent, global action, we risk going back to a pre-antibiotic era; with collaboration and innovation, we can ensure that future generations can access the treatments they need.

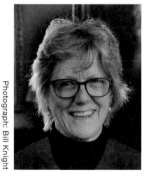

Photograph: Bill Knight

Dame Sally Davies FRS is the 40th Master of Trinity College, University of Cambridge and the UK Government's Special Envoy on Antimicrobial Resistance (AMR). From 2011–2019, she was Chief Medical Officer for England and Chief Medical Adviser to the UK Government. Dame Sally is a member of the UN Global Leaders Group on AMR, since 2020. Fellow of the Royal Society and Member of the US National Academy of Science. Awarded both DBE and GCB.

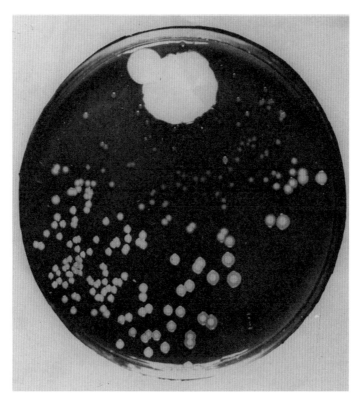

Photograph of the original culture plate of the fungus *Penicillium notatum* made by Sir Alexander Fleming while working at St. Mary's Hospital, Paddington, London. Courtesy of the Alexander Fleming Laboratory Museum, Imperial College Healthcare NHS Trust

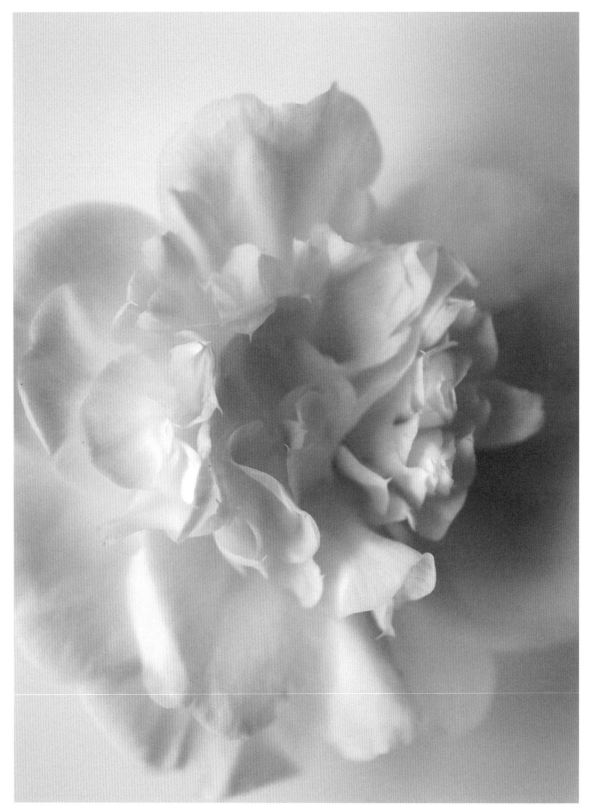

Blooming

Carole Collet
DESIGN RESEARCHER

When one is said to be 'blooming', this entails a notion of flourishment, vitality, and a picture of health that is both physical and mental. I chose to create a photograph of a seasonal Camelia bloom to evoke the notion of 'blooming' with nested narratives. Human health is inherently connected to the plant world. The oxygen we intake is produced by the plant world around us and our well-being as a species is deeply inter-twinned with planetary health. The 3.8 billion-year-old plant biodiversity we have inherited provides a wide range of medicines and benefits, yet it is a world threatened by our activities. Today, we are in the midst of a rapid human-induced biodiversity collapse, so with this image, I wanted to remind us that our health is deeply interconnected with the 'tangled banks' of other species as described by Charles Darwin and that we should value each and every bloom. The resilience of the natural world is often confronted by its fragility. I created a portrait of a white flower which is easily bruised to offer a hint into a biological materiality of infinite intricacies and constantly evolving genetic possibilities as a symbol of our fragile health.

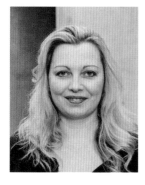

Professor Carole Collet, Central Saint Martins University of the Arts London, is co-director of the Living Systems Lab, set up in 2013 as a pioneering research group to explore living systems thinking for the pursuit of new ecological knowledge in the creative sector. She is also Director of Maison/0, a platform for regenerative luxury co-developed with the luxury group LVMH to leverage creativity at the service of ecosystem regeneration. She is recognised for her leadership in ecological design centered on biodesign and biomimicry principles. She regularly contributes to international conferences and publications on the subjects of living systems design, biodesign, and regenerative futures.

Robert Gallo
VIROLOGIST

In 1984, we published this figure (top right) in a paper in the journal *Science*. It was the first time that the well-established laboratory research technique known as 'western blotting' had been employed in a clinical diagnostic setting. This result was key confirmation that HIV caused AIDS. Needless to say, the blood test saved the blood supply of the world, preventing HIV infections by medical use of blood and plasma. It also allowed the pandemic to be followed for the first time – before, one had to wait until a patient showed signs of AIDS which was many months or even years. Finally, it was an easy, cheap test and was used globally to link HIV to AIDS causatively. Establishing the blood test for global use also demanded massive virus production, technology we invented, growing HIV in a continuous cell line culture, which also enabled the test for and finding of the first successful anti-virus (of any kind) drugs for a systemic virus disease in medical history.

My team in 1984 (lower right) is a prime example of a picture of health. Women and men, intelligent, passionate about their work and all in the prime of their life (with the exception of the very fortunate Lab Head).

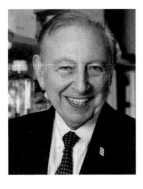

Homer & Martha Gudelsky Distinguished Professor in Medicine and Microbiology, Robert Gallo studied medicine at Thomas Jefferson University, Yale, and Chicago University. Working for 30 years at the National Cancer Institute of the National Institutes of Health (NIH), he and his colleagues discovered the first cytokine, IL-2; the first pathogenic human retroviruses, including HTLV-1, one of the first human cancer viruses; co-discovered HIV as the cause of AIDS and developed the HIV blood test. In 1996 he co-founded the Institute of Human Virology at the University of Maryland School of Medicine and, in 2011, the Global Virus Network, where he is Scientific International Advisor.

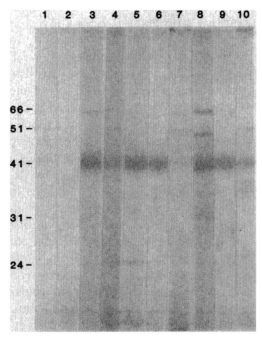

Image from Sarngadharan et al, *Science*, May 1984

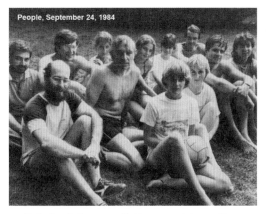

Gallo (centre) poses with his research team after a
competitive round of volleyball during their weekly
Sunday gathering at his home near the NIH in
September 1984

Photograph: Clive Thompson

Freewheelers
THEATRE COMPANY

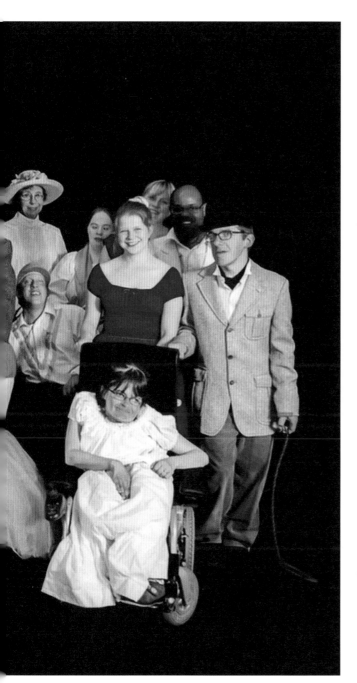

With locations across Surrey, we make theatre, dance, film, music and visual art that challenge perceptions and defies expectations.

Working alongside professional arts practitioners, every week is packed with creative workshops where members come together to co-create and share their creative talents, learn new skills and work towards a new performance, film or piece of art.

This photo is of the company in costume for the stage production of 'Degas' – the story of the life of the painter told in dance, music, drama and art.

Founded over thirty years ago The Freewheelers Theatre Company has been a force of change and artistic excellence in the world of Disability Art.

Karen Sarkisyan

SYNTHETIC BIOLOGIST

Healthcare is fuelled by technologies, and technologies stem from basic research. Our bioluminescence project was started by our colleagues as purely basic research and has developed into technology to create tissues and organisms that report their physiology by glowing in the dark. We hope that this technology will form the basis for the next generation of bioluminescence tools to be used in a variety of medical research – from monitoring cancer development to visualising pathological states – as well as in diagnostics, synthetic biology and agriculture.

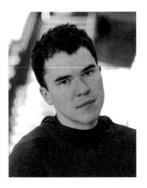

The Sarkisyan lab focuses on developing new molecular technologies and applying them to study biology. Before starting the lab at the LMS, Karen worked on fluorescent protein development with Konstantin Lukyanov and Alexander Mishin in Moscow, and then studied protein evolution with Fyodor Kondrashov in Barcelona and Vienna.

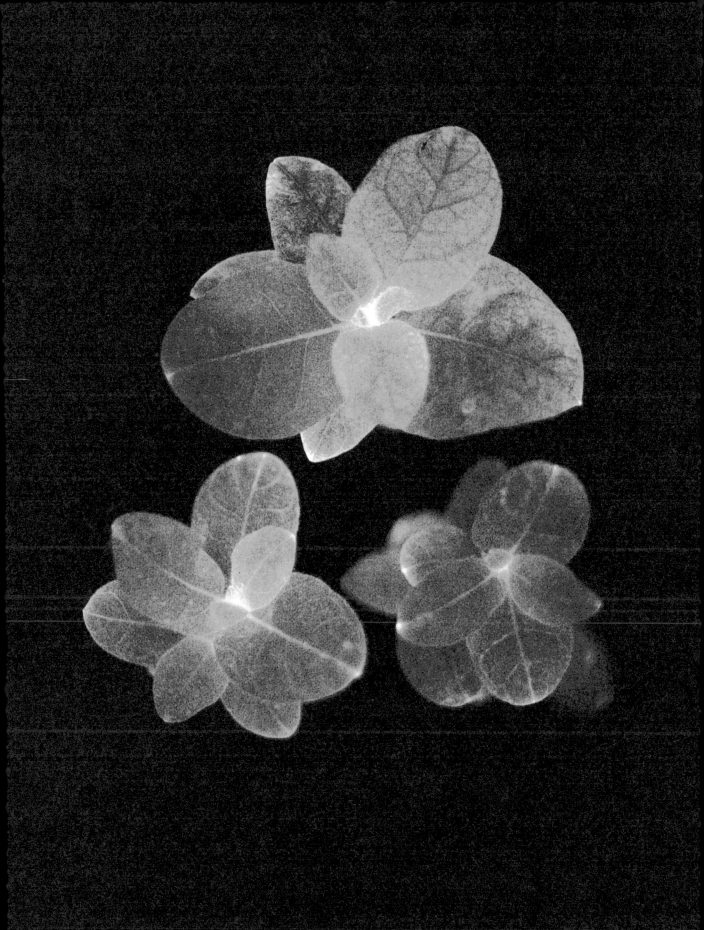

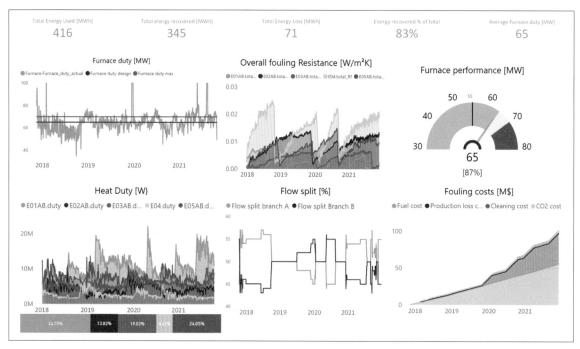

The indicators show that this plant is healthy, productive, energy efficient and environmentally friendly

Francesco Coletti

CHEMICAL ENGINEER

Industrial plants use energy to convert raw materials into useful products. The health of industrial systems is directly related to our own: a healthy plant produces useful materials that increase our living standards, uses resources efficiently and has minimal impact on our environment.

Unlike human health, the health of industrial equipment can be accurately measured and predicted into the future using digital twins: mathematical representations of the plant that allow us to use real time measurements from the plant itself to assess the health of the equipment, the environmental and economic impact of operations and diagnose causes of faults or bad performance. They also allow us to predict when issues might occur, thus helping prevent them and keeping the equipment healthy and efficient. The picture shows various indicators of the thermal performance of a chemical plant, including amount of energy used, the amount of deposits impairing efficiency, performance of the furnace and the cumulative costs of operations.

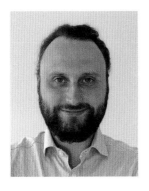

Dr. Francesco Coletti is a Chemical Engineer and the CEO of Hexxcell Ltd., a London based technology company providing predictive analytics and prescriptive maintenance solutions for industrial heat transfer systems. He is also a part-time Associate Professor at Brunel University London where he contributed to the launch of a new Chemical Engineering Department.

Frank Close

PARTICLE PHYSICIST

As any follower of Star Trek knows when matter meets its opposite – antimatter – they mutually annihilate. The simplest example of antimatter is the positron, the anti-particle of the humble electron. Electrons are present in the atoms and molecules of everything, including the human body.

Some radioactive materials emit positrons. This is key to the PET scanner in medical diagnostics. PET stands for positron emission tomography. Positrons emitted by an appropriate radioactive nucleus, which the patient has ingested, will annihilate with electrons close by and produce gamma rays. The gamma rays can be detected and from this an image of the distribution of chemicals in the brain or elsewhere in the body obtained.

The annihilation of positrons is an important diagnostic tool in medicine that is saving lives every day. The fundamental annihilation of an electron by a positron is a standard process in particle physics, and the resulting images provide beautiful pieces of art work. This is literally a picture of health.

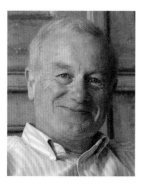

Frank Close, OBE FRS is Emeritus Professor of Theoretical Physics and Fellow of Exeter College at the University of Oxford. In 1975 he joined the Rutherford Appleton Laboratory in Oxfordshire as a research particle physicist, becoming head of the Theoretical Physics Division in 1991. After leading public education at CERN, he became Professor of Theoretical Physics at Oxford in 2001. His many awards for the popularisation of science include the Royal Society's Michael Faraday Prize for Science Communication, and his books include the highly acclaimed history of particle physics, The Infinity Puzzle, *and the latest* Elusive, *a biography of Higgs' boson.*

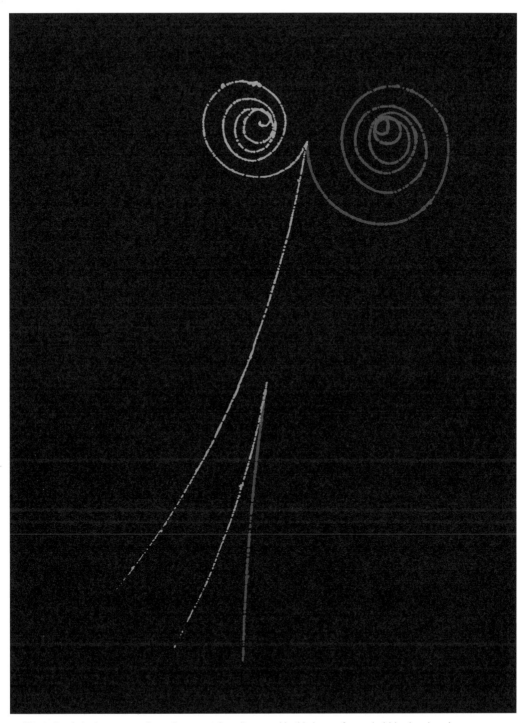

The trails of electrons are coloured green and positrons red in this image from a bubble chamber. A gamma ray has knocked an electron from an atom at the top, but has enough residual energy to convert into an electron and positron. In a PET scanner, this happens in reverse: the electron and positron annihilate into photons.
Photograph: Science Photo Library

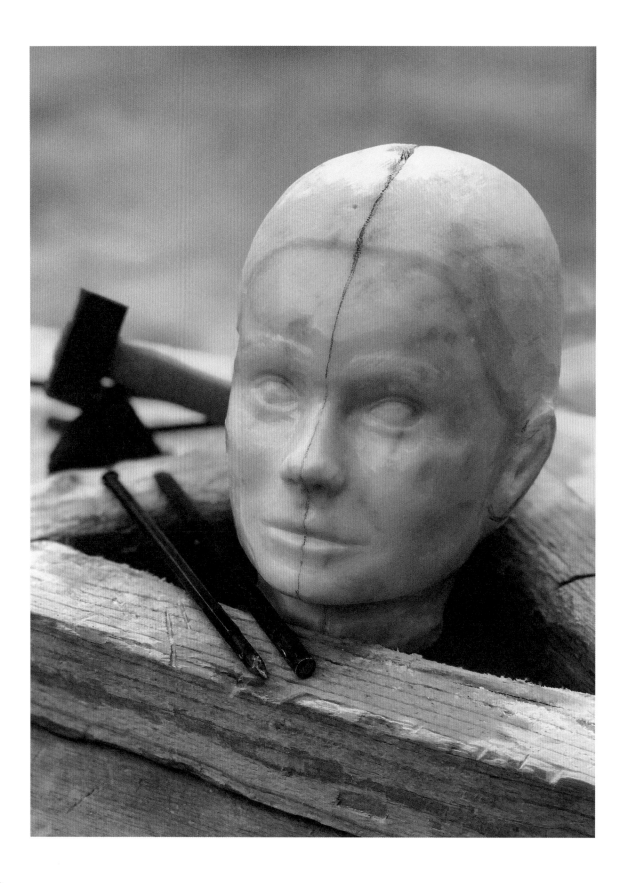

Mandel von Glasow

CONTEMPORARY JEWELLER AND ARTIST

It took me a long time to think about what my picture of health would be. I have an enormous passion for agriculture and ecology, so at first I was thinking about how to represent our life-giving planet as a jewellery object. But my idea felt forced and generic. Especially because we all, mostly unthinking and unapologetically work against the health of our planet. Then as I often do I thought about a disagreement I had with a dear friend a few years ago. I started to carve her portrait, and over the weeks that I was chiselling away it gave me plenty of time to reflect upon what I would've done differently and how I can improve myself to not repeat the same mistakes again. The process of making this marble sculpture helped me greatly reflect on what I can do better. So, this piece became my picture of health.

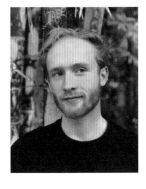

Mandel von Glasow was born in London where he also completed his secondary education. He graduated the BFA Class of 2021 at Alchimia Contemporary Jewellery Academy in Firenze and is now a budding Florence based contemporary jeweller and artist.

John Biltcliffe
FILM MAKER

During lockdown, I found myself daydreaming about the places I wanted to see and it frustrated me waking up to the same things everyday. I took this feeling and went an extra step with it, imagining waking up and seeing the same room everyday, as a hospitalised person does. I would daydream considerably more. The video ended up being a visualisation of this, with the flashing lights representing the days passing in the outside world and the locations being the places that I was daydreaming about. My first ideas for this project always contained dance as it is such a clear display of physical health. This is something that naturally comes with fantasies. I also thought, "Why not try and get as many different artistic practices in as I can?". Music, dance and film.

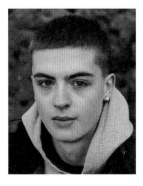

John Biltcliffe is a 19-year-old filmmaker currently studying at The Northern Film School who started his film education five years ago at the BRIT School. His passion for film has been around as long as he can remember. He has won awards for his work at a number of short film festivals.

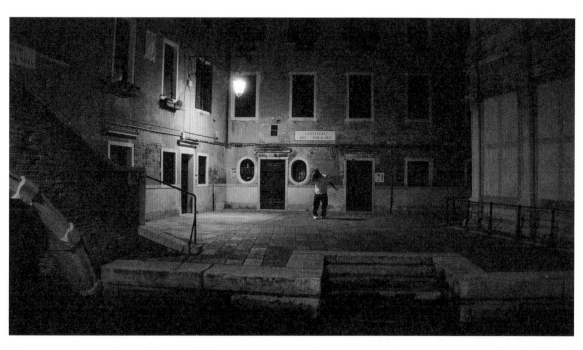

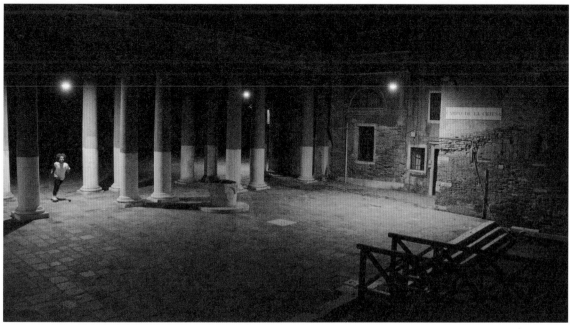

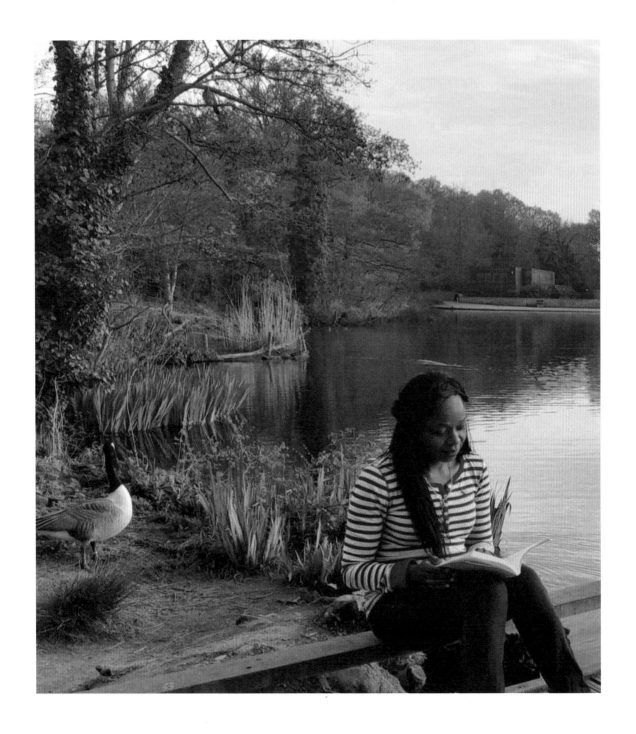

Lydia Noa

TRAINING CENTRE MANAGER

Reading in the park for me, is a form of relaxation, in a quiet place, on a bench where there is little noise and all that matters is my connection with the book I am reading. I have acquired this habit during the lockdown; as I was spending a long period of time working, I felt that I needed to have something to help me relax when I was tired. When COVID-19 restrictions eased a little and we gradually went out of lockdown, I found myself wanting to keep this habit. My favourite spot to read is on a small bench, overlooking a pond with a family of white swans that constantly increases in number. It is a great opportunity to think about what I am reading, how it makes me feel, or simply enjoy the nature around me. It can be any novel – mystery, drama, comedy – I do not mind, just something I can read for around an hour without getting bored. Generally, I enjoy reading in any environment, especially at home, but there are many distractions; noise coming from the television, a family member speaking loudly, or someone requesting me to do something, which is why I normally opt for the park.

Overall, reading in the park is a great way to clear my mind, be alone with my thoughts and of course, enjoy the book! I often find it therapeutic and definitely recommend this to others.

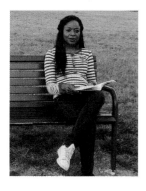

Lydia Noa is the manager of the UKRI Engineering and Physical Sciences Research Council's Centre for Doctoral Training in Mathematics of Random Systems. She joined the department of Mathematics at Imperial College in June 2019. She previously worked at Imperial College as a Grants administrator within the Joint Research Office and as a Research Group Administrator at the National Heart & Lung Institute, prior to that she worked at the MRC supporting research groups.

Suzanne Iwai
AUTISTIC ACTIVIST

With my poetry, my aim is to show other people who have shielded during the pandemic, have ever suffered from feeling marginalised or isolated, that being healthy is achievable through a creative outlet. A picture of health can be a mandala, a mindmap, a drawing, a piece of knitting or crochet, a jigsaw, a quilt, a homemade birthday card, a tray of cupcakes shared with a friend, a song sung together or over the phone, a joke you can't stop laughing at even though you've heard it before, some silliness you see your grandchild do, and in my case, it's sitting absorbed in writing a poem with a smile on my face.

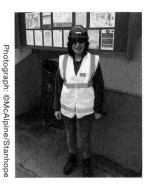

Photograph: ©McAlpine/Stanhope

Living on White City Estate since 1999, I am vice chair of WC Residents' Association, also an Agent of Change a women's equality, inclusion and diversity network, and a Disabled Co-producer with the London Borough of Hammersmith & Fulham. Helping deliver autistic support differently as a late life diagnosed person, I do citizen scientist research with Autistica and patient participation with Voice Global. I enjoy writing poetry (under my pseudonym Suzi Qpid) and plan to publish a booklet of In the Years of Covid poems. I am a lively book in the Human Library a global peace/ diversity organisation and a member of the Bush Theatre Neighbourhood company.

Less Slug… more?

In Wisdom fusion we're all sweetly sharpened tools
Firmly declaring we're no one else's fool
Stretching into and exploring repurposed versions of ourselves
No one is left on dusty and abandoned shaky shelves.

We're shedding the musty, no longer needed masks
From our individual and collective pasts
Gazing into the mirror of reflected experiences
Do you recognise the person staring back at you?
Is it a made up image or is it authentic and true.

What does that even mean… sounds simple, squeaky clean

Do you show up to fulfill your own needs
Or contribute to other peoples' newsfeed?

Me… I'm striving to be elastic
Wouldn't that be fantastic…
Crawling like an amorphous slug
Across a great expanse of infinite white
A curiously contracting glistening grimy grey
Yet boldly and confidently making its way
Into a space where it can expand into
Whatever happens next.
Be that small, medium or super grand.

Size or speed doesn't matter in any of this
It's focusing on fluidity and the flow
Of possibilities none of which can be missed
Every opportunity expertly super fished.
HELL the cells in your body change all the time
The slug sheds parts of itself as it slides in its slime.

So if you decide growing is existentially essentially YOU…
BECOME THE CHANGE YOU WISH TO SEE
At your pace, no starting gun, no race,
No pressure to do, to do, TO DO.
With patience and grace, I'm less Slug
I'm morphing into a GLOWWORM State of Being.

Hunt Emerson
COMICS ARTIST AND CARTOONIST

I have practiced Tai Chi for about 20 years, and until recently I was a qualified Tai Chi instructor. The Gentle Martial Art is a great promoter of, and aid to general health and well-being. I recommend it to anyone who asks. My comic strip hints at a few of the moves in the Tai Chi Form, but it is meant to be a lampoon. One does not usually lose one's trousers while doing Tai Chi. The "I don't do stress…" motto is from my Tai Chi teacher Mark Peters, but I endorse it wholeheartedly!

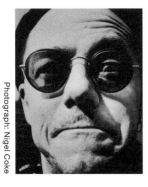

Photograph: Nigel Coke

Born in Newcastle in 1952, and resident in Birmingham since the early 1970s, Hunt Emerson has drawn comics for over 40 years. He has published more than 30 books of his iconoclastic comic strips, including The Cartoon Lady Chatterley's Lover, The Rime of the Ancient Mariner, Casanova's Last Stand, Dante's Inferno, *and most recently,* Lives of the Great Occultists *and* Phenomenomix. *In 2000 Hunt was chosen for inclusion in the exhibition 75 Masters of European Comic Art by the Bibliotheque Nationale de France and the Cité Internationale de la Bande Dessinnée et de l'Image, Angouleme. In 2018 he was given a Sergio Award (named after Sergio Aragonés) by the National Cartoonists Society of America.*

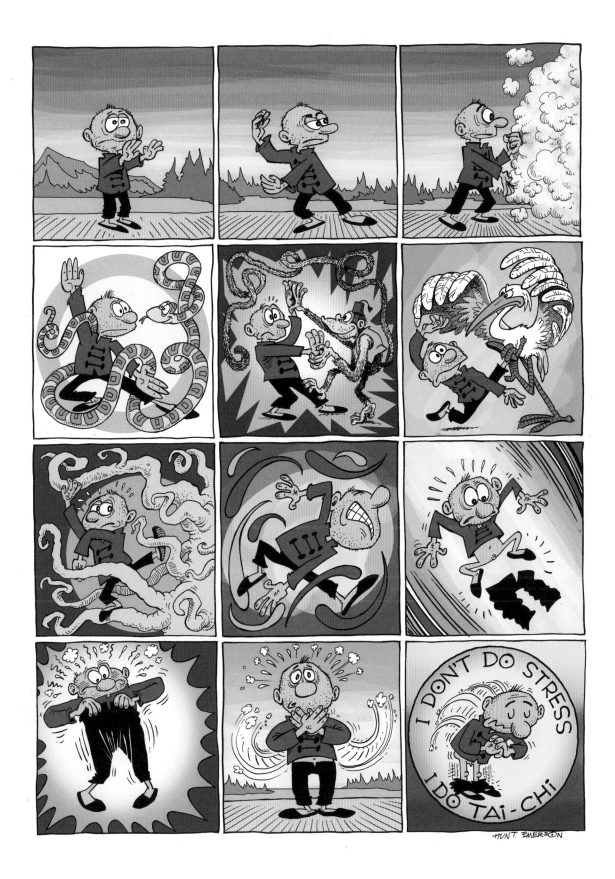

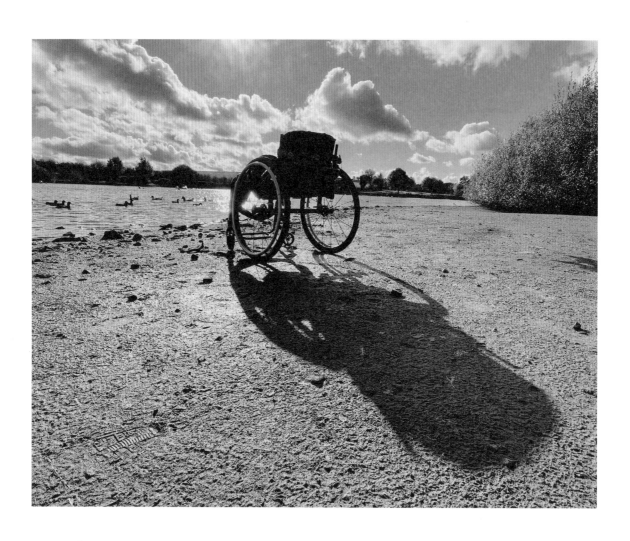

Susan Whitfield
MOTIVATIONAL SPEAKER

Losing health is massive. A life changing event. It affects every part of
   you: your head, your heart, even how you pay the rent.
It knocks the health of others – fells them like big trees. There's nothing
   you can do to help as you're ground down to your knees.

There're lumps, bumps and boulders and things I can't get over.
Twist and turns that throw me, the people that look through me.
The 'if nots', 'can nots', 'should nots'; the list of body shall nots.
The views, the smiles, the head shakes, they're things you can't mistake.

But I find the silver lining, the reason to keep being me because it's not
   defining – well it's not defining me!

The calm, the still, the open, that makes me feel unbroken.
The rhythm, speed and beauty, the people that look to me.
The can do, want to, able to; the body that enables you.
The view, the smile, the head space, the feelings that it creates.

I have found a way of being free and, most importantly, I've found the
   new me.

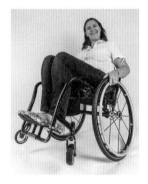

In 2008 I was a fit paramedic. Then my world was shattered with a progressive neurological condition diagnosis. Slowly the list of things I was unable to do grew. Being unable to do the basic human functions is hard to come to terms with. As a full-time wheelchair user people see me as disabled, unable, unwell, even unworthy. Nine years later I was diagnosed with leukaemia which it seemed wanted to kill me quicker! 'Unable' just got cellular! Then I re-found swimming, and due to the pandemic, open-water swimming. A true silver lining! A priceless getaway from the restraints of my broken body. A freedom like no other.

Catherine Denvir

ARTIST

My first ever swim in the pinky, brown or sometimes greeny blue grey English Channel instilled in me a lifelong love of swimming and the sea.

Swimming with my mother at Kenwood Ladies' Pond, on Hampstead Heath, an exotic secret garden of a place in my memory an Arcadia compared to the municipal swimming pools and lidos of south London, not that those places didn't have a charm of their own.

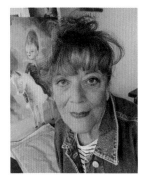

Catherine Denvir studied at Chelsea School of Art and went on to become a prolific illustrator working for magazines, publishers and advertising mainly in the UK but also France, Germany and the USA. Clients include Penguin Books, Random House, Vogue, New Scientist *and* Adobe. *Catherine now paints full time, her work selling to collectors in the United States, Canada, Italy, the UK and Germany.*

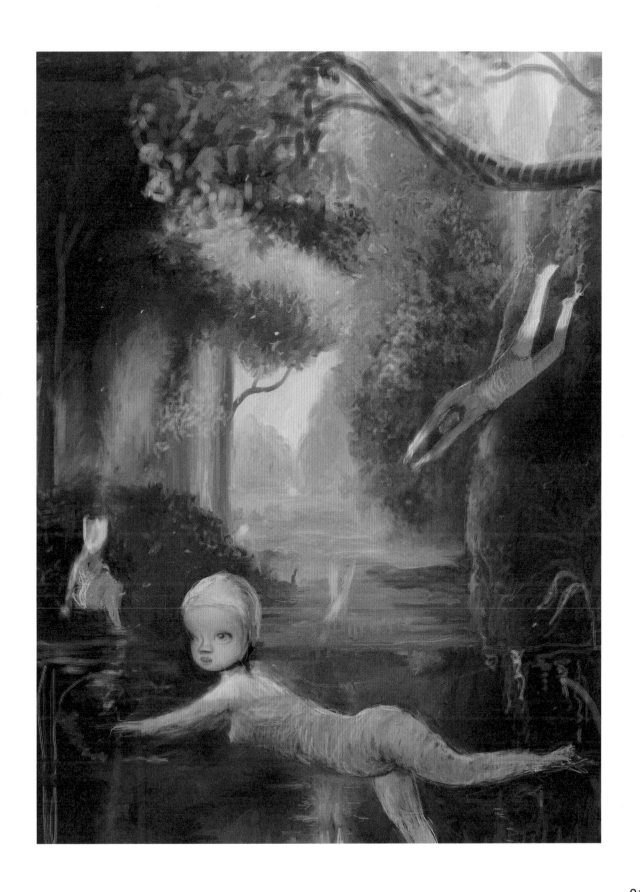

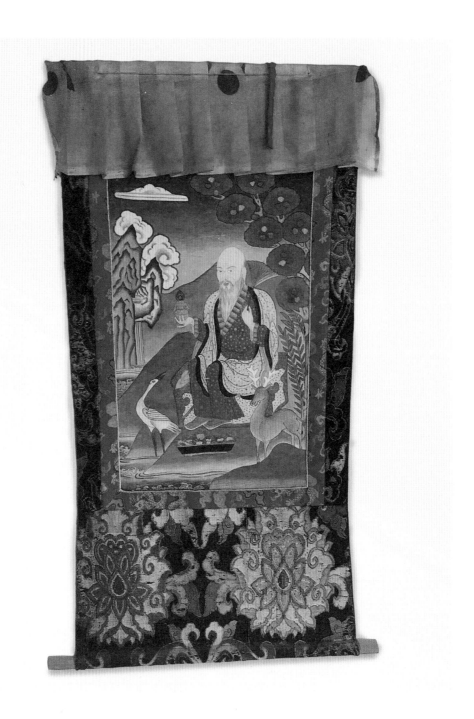

Ringu Tulku Rinpoche

TIBETAN LAMA

Hearing the words *A Picture of Health* the first thought that came to me was Tsering Namdruk (Six Symbols of Long Life). This is a drawing or a painting we have in every Tibetan house usually. This picture is painted either as a thanka scroll or on the wall of a house. It is said that if you keep this painting in your house it will bring long life and health and harmony to the family living there. We have a small painting hanging in the entrance of my room above the staircase. This is painted by my brother when he was a student of thanka painting.

Six Symbols of Long Life:
Long Life Deer, Long Life Rock, Long Life River, Long Life Bird, Long Life Tree and Long life Man

On the slope of long life Rocky mountain,
Sleeps peacefully the long life deer with ten horns.
Besides the long life river of pure spring
Freely walks the long life storks.
Under the leafy branches of long life tree.
Happily relaxes the long living elderly hermit.

Besides, there are Buddha of Immeasurable Life and Medicine Buddha, White Tara and other health- and life-giving deities. There are also humans like Guru Padma Sambhava and Lady Mandarava who are known to have attained immortality. There are also various practices and trainings how to attain this, which anyone can practice.

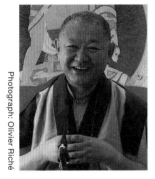

Photograph: Olivier Riché

Ringu Tulku Rinpoche is a monk and a Tibetan Buddhist Master of the Kagyu Order. His training included all four major schools of Tibetan Buddhism. Among his teachers were HH the 16th Gyalwang Karmapa and HH Dilgo Khentse Rinpoche. He was born in 1952 and fled with his family between 1957 and 1959 from Tibet to India. Since then he has lived in Sikkim. He has been teaching Buddhism and meditation all over the world since 1990. He wrote several books on Buddhism and founded several organizations to promote Buddhist teachings and intercultural dialogues.

Virginia Bottomley

FORMER HEALTH MINISTER

Swimming has always been my primary life-enhancing and re-energising activity. From a young age I competed actively in a local swimming club.

Now, as Baroness Bottomley of Nettlestone, our home faces beautiful Priory Bay. Our grandchildren play there as the fifth generation in our family. Our great-uncles and aunts started the tradition of swimming to St Helen's Fort, a Napoleonic fort in the Solent. They mastered the challenge at 18 and my father at 16. I broke the record aged 10 in swimming this mile-long journey. Our children swam at eight. The Fort swim has become a rite of passage.

During my time as Cabinet Minister responsible for the NHS, I introduced the first 'Health of the Nation' strategy in the early '90s. It was commended by the Organisation for Economic Co-operation and Development but condemned as 'too nannying' by political colleagues. This strategy has stood the test of time. Behaviour change, prevention, good diet and above all exercise can do so much to enhance physical and mental well-being. As the years progress, we all understand this better and there is evidence to prove it.

Today a group of Isle of Wight swimmers, Swim the Wight, offer community involvement in the life-enhancing activity of open water swimming – companionship in water temperatures varying from 20°C in summer to 6°C in winter.

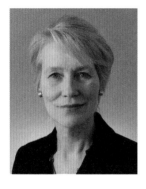

Virginia held several Ministerial positions under Baroness Margaret Thatcher and Sir John Major. A junior Environment Minister in 1987, she became Minister for Health from 1989–92 and Secretary of State for Health from 1992–95. From 1995–97 she was the Secretary of State for Culture, Media and Sport. In 2005 she was appointed a member of the House of Lords taking the title Rt Hon Baroness Bottomley of Nettlestone DL. Following her first degree, Virginia gained her MSc in Social Administration from the London School of Economics.

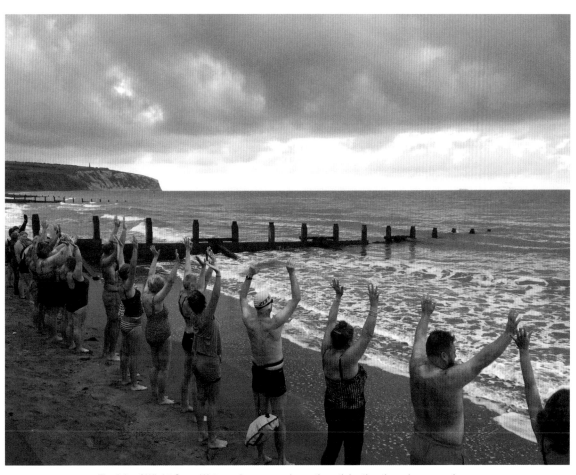

The Isle of Wight Open Water swimmers exuberantly anticipating the unique experience and benefits offered by submersion in the water. Photograph: Perdita Hunt

Willy Russell
PLAYWRIGHT

Common or Garden

A common or garden plant – something one would expect to find on common land, open field or uncultivated garden.

We scattered some seeds, a random mix on the barren patch, covered them over with the cold, damp January soil. We supposed that not much would come of our admittedly meagre efforts and by the time the March winds blew, our planting was mostly forgotten. And then the air softened, the days grew warmer and green shoots appeared, straining for the sky, swelling with the April showers; and bursting, exploding their glory into the warm May sun.

Time to get out the inks, the brushes, the paint, the paper and canvas; time to try and catch and hold something of this patch of unremarkable treasure, this all too common or garden miracle. Time. It won't always be spring.

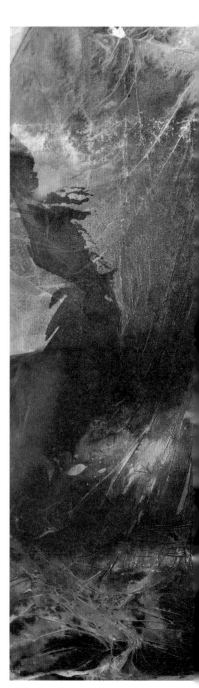

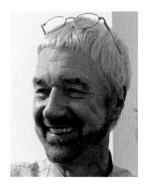

Willy Russell is a multi-award-winning playwright and Oscar-nominated screenwriter. Works such as Educating Rita, Shirley Valentine, *and the musical,* Blood Brothers *have become modern classics constantly in production on the British stage and throughout the world. Russell has* always explored and experimented with other associated art forms, achieving considerable success as a composer, lyricist, novelist and (occasional) performer. *In recent years he has become an enthusiastic student of the visual arts, developing his skills as a printmaker and painter.*

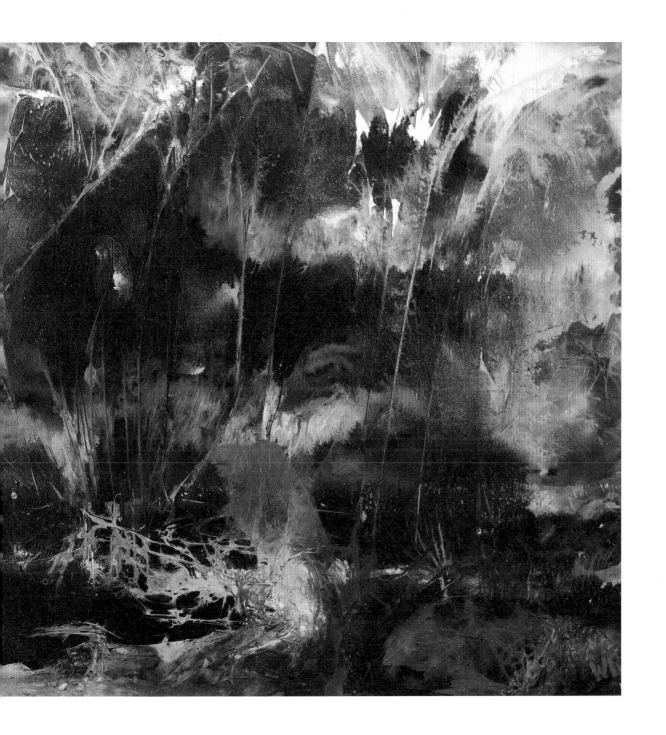

Elisha Gabb

POET

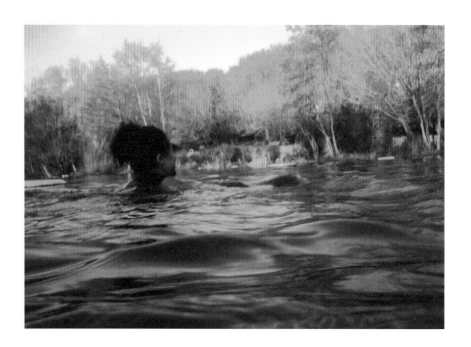

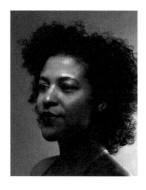

Elisha Gabb is a mixed-race writer from London who is currently doing a Creative Writing MA at Brunel University. As a teenager Elisha travelled around the world representing Great Britain as a junior tennis player. Her travels inspire her writing today and her short story My Home in Transit *was recently published in* Litro Magazine. *She also enjoys writing and performing her poetry. She is currently finalising her first novel. When Elisha isn't writing you'll find her swimming in the Hampstead Heath ponds, meditating, or dancing the night away with her friends.*

Nirvana

I see her
Holding her space so beautifully amongst the naked wilderness
That sculps itself around her oval belly
White mist rises as she exhales towards the morning sky
She welcomes us

Bare bodied with a bit of cloth covering my core
I stare at her, excitement and fear
Overlap one another racing for first place
But before either of them have a chance to win
Gently she pulls me in

I join her in exhaling loudly so she can hear me
My first few strokes are almost unbearable
Her honesty burns my skin, but I know I need to feel it
A quarter of the way round she softens on my body
As she begins to wash my mind

Swallowing yesterday's terrors, she tells me all I need to know
I think of nothing
The trees swoop lower to greet her, and then to greet me
I smile, I look around at the other bodies
We're all ok

I wonder if she knows she heals us
That her coldness fills our hearts with so much warmth
Arise and cease she stays

She's a woman and her name is Water

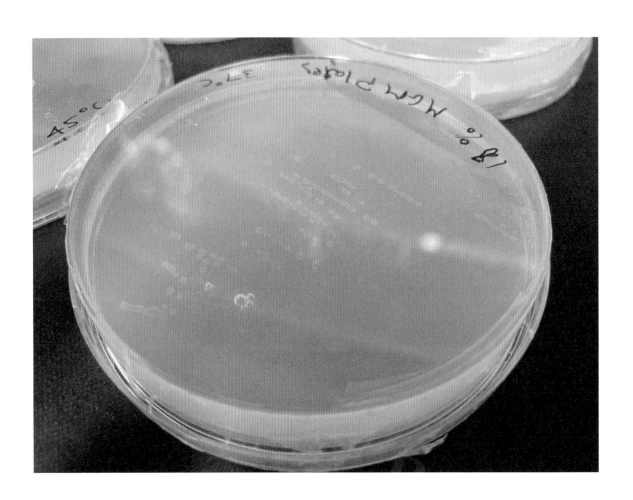

Tobias Warnecke
EVOLUTIONARY BIOLOGIST

We work on archaea – tiny single-celled organisms not unlike bacteria but with a molecular toolkit that, in many respects, is more similar to that of humans. Some of these archaea flourish in odd places. The bright pink *Haloferax volcanii* colonies in this picture, for example, were originally isolated from the Dead Sea. They love extremely salty environments where few other organisms survive. Other archaea thrive closer to home: in the human gut. Here, they have carved out a living for themselves amongst legions of bacteria. We study how these archaea defend themselves against bacterial competitors, looking for new types of antibacterial molecules that can be used to combat antimicrobial resistance. This is my picture of health as it reminds me that solutions to health challenges, now and in the future, can come from the strangest of places.

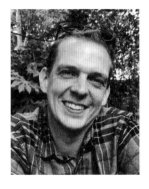

Dr Tobias Warnecke is an MRC Investigator at the LMS. His group works on how very different organisms – from predatory bacteria to humans – compact and organise their DNA. He has a particular interest in archaea, microorganisms that can be found in many different places – the sea, the soil, and the digestive tract of humans – but whose intimate interactions with other microbes, as well as their human host, remain enigmatic.

Joanna Parr
GEOLOGIST

Geology seeks to give us a fundamental understanding of how our planet 'works' and is pivotal to our well-being. As geologists we work as part of multidisciplinary teams that explore the interface between humans and the planet, looking for solutions to current and anticipated societal challenges and giving context to the impacts humans have on our habitable zone.

With my colleagues I have been exploring the seafloor for over 30 years. Two thirds of the Earth is covered by oceans, hiding mountain ranges, active volcanoes and vast abyssal plains and yet only a tiny fraction has been explored and investigated. Around seafloor volcanoes, vents of hot waters up to 400°C, charged with dissolved gases and minerals, emerge through fractures onto the seafloor and form 'fields' – like these in the eastern Bismarck Sea in Papua New Guinea – of chimney-like structures rich in metals including iron, zinc, copper and occasionally gold, providing natural laboratories that help us understand how mineral deposits formed millions of years ago. They are also amazing oases of life surviving in extreme conditions – crabs, worms, snails, shrimp and other creatures, specialised at living at great depths and pressures and in complete darkness. Below the seafloor, the marine sediments contain evidence about the health of the oceans through time. In particular, changes that have driven the abundance, diversity, and recovery of life following mass extinctions.

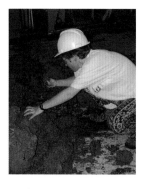

Dr Joanna Parr is Executive Manager of Operations for the Mineral Resources Business Unit in Australia's Commonwealth Science and Industry Research Organisation (CSIRO). She was President (2018–2021) of the Geological Society of Australia and a lead member of the International Ocean Discovery Program – Australia-New Zealand Consortium. Following study of 1.8 billion-year-old rocks in Sweden and Australia, she joined the CSIRO team studying active geological processes on the SW Pacific Ocean floor. The team discovered multiple major hydrothermally venting sites and triggered an important new area of research and discovery. In 2002 they received CSIRO's most prestigious Chairman's Medal for their pioneering research.

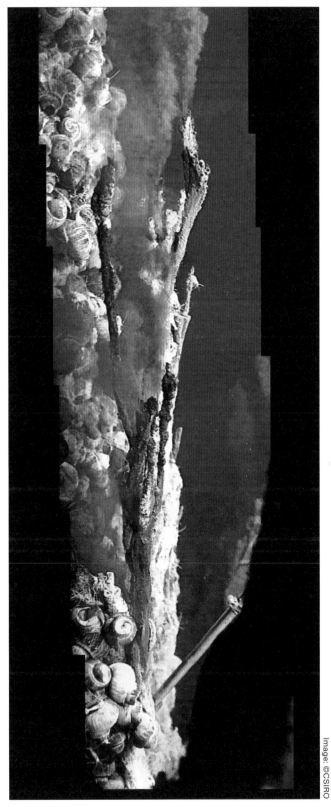

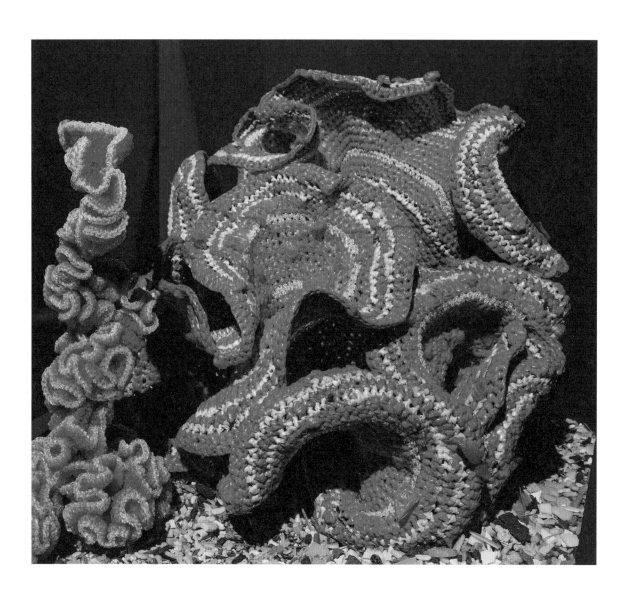

Margaret Wertheim

SCIENCE WRITER ARTIST

Science writer and artist Margaret Wertheim's work focuses on relations between science and the wider cultural landscape. Author of six books, including a trilogy about the history of physics, her writing has appeared in the New York Times, Los Angeles Times, Guardian, Cabinet, *and* Aeon. *With her sister Christine, she co-founded the Institute For Figuring, devoted to the aesthetic dimensions of science, through which they have created exhibits for many international venues. The sisters' Crochet Coral Reef is a worldwide science+art project that has been exhibited at the 2019 Venice Biennale, 2021 Helsinki Biennial and other international venues. Margaret's reef TED Talk has been viewed over 1.5 million times.*

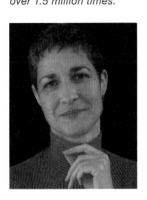

The Crochet Reef began in 2005, when – in response to devastation on the Great Barrier Reef in their native state of Queensland – the sisters Margaret and Christine Wertheim conceived of constructing an artificial reef, based on the fact that corals, kelps and other sea creatures are biological incarnations of *hyperbolic* geometry, an alternative to the usual Euclidean variety.

Through an unlikely fusion of mathematics, marine biology, handicraft and collective art practice, the Wertheims and their contributors produce large-scale coralline landscapes both beautiful and blighted. The Crochet Coral Reef offers a beautiful impassioned response to dual calamities devastating marine life: climate change and plastic trash.

Each crochet 'species' is descended from the simple seeds of a mathematically pure hyperbolic crochet surface discovered by Cornell mathematician Dr. Daina Taimina. By morphing and complexifying an underlying code – the pattern of crochet stitches – a dynamically unfolding, wooly 'tree of life' has been brought into being. In this marriage of mathematical experimentation and material play the Crochet Coral Reef constitutes a novel alliance between science and art characterized by process, development, and open-mindedness; here, the art-making itself recapitulates processes at the heart of organic evolution. Art becomes a tool not just for learning about science, but for enacting methodologies within nature that science uncovers.

By inviting in people from all walks of life – scientists, housewives, teachers, computer programmers, sheep farmers, prisoners, and shelter residents among them – the Crochet Coral Reef offers a radical alternative to the model of artist as singular prodigy. Just as living reefs result from collaboration between billions of coral polyps who collectively construct such marvels as the Great Barrier Reef, so crocheted Satellite Reefs embody the creative potential of crowds.

Nicholas J.P. Owens

MARINE SCIENTIST

My picture of health is about the health of the oceans. This image of a humpback whale gives me hope. It suggests that we are on the way back to a world whose seas are full of whales. This would return us to the plentiful time before we humans began whale hunting, in the 18th century, to the time before the industrial-scale slaughter that existed right up to the mid-20th century. Sadly, whales are still killed, though in much smaller numbers. And we are well on the way to a reset: nearly every study shows increasing populations everywhere. Whales are long-lived animals, with lifespans that are similar to humans. It will take time to rebuild populations from near extinction. Yes, we really did nearly do this. So, my chosen image depicts not only the health of the ocean, but also the hope that we are beginning to realise our responsibility, to adopt a humble position on this planet. This image is also one of fun: this humpback whale is having a 'whale of a time'.

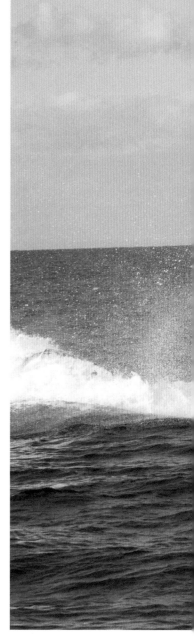

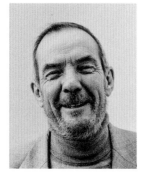

Professor Nicholas Owens is the Executive Director of the Scottish Association for Marine Science (SAMS), which is based in Oban, on the West coast of Scotland. He is a marine scientist and has written over 130 scientific publications in marine biogeochemistry. He has spent around five years of his life at sea, on research vessels, on all the oceans of the planet. He is a former Director of several research institutes, including the British Antarctic Survey.

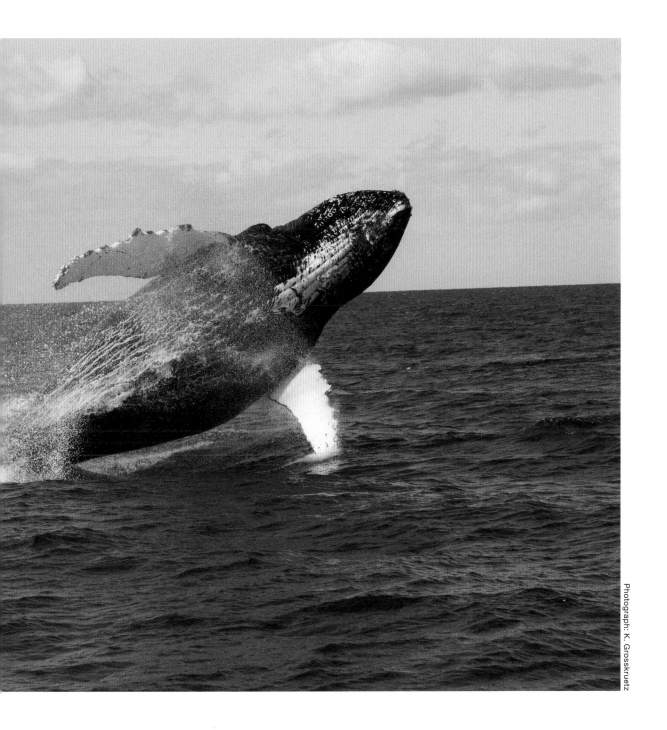

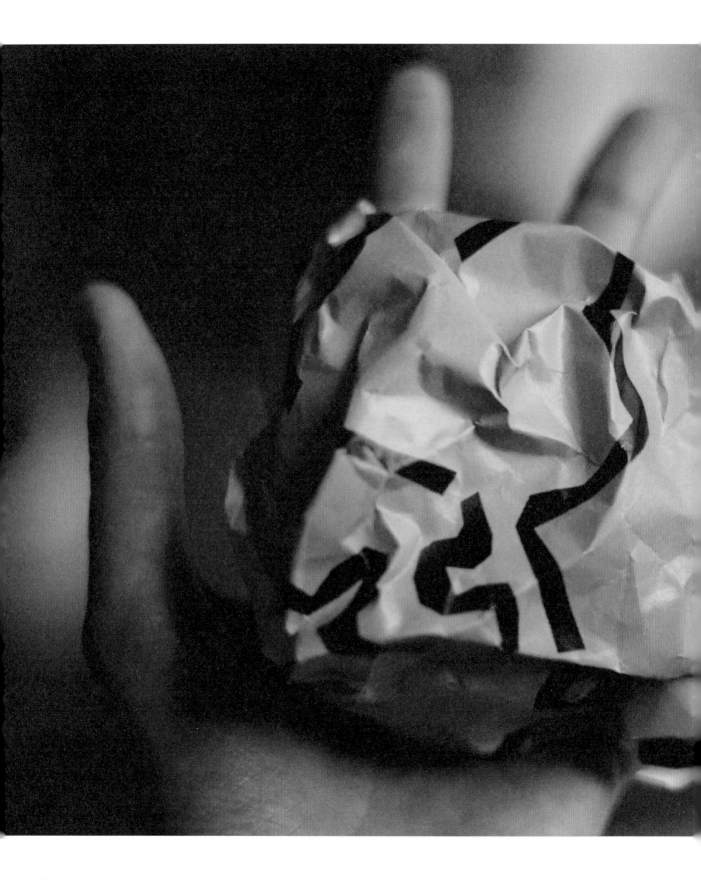

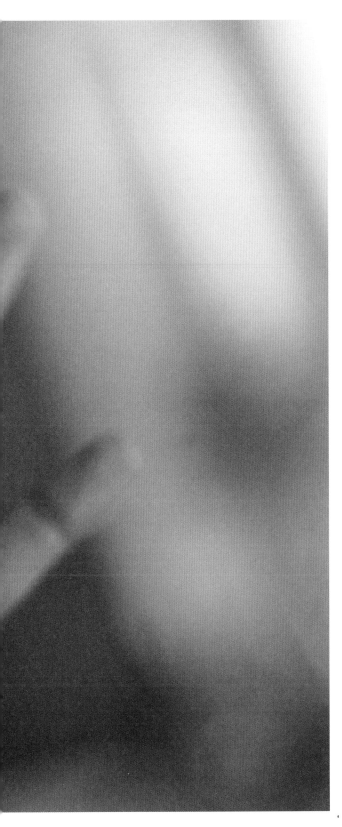

Greening LMS
RECYCLING GROUP

Much of what we do as scientists is to make the world a better place but the practice of generating reliable research often results in a considerable amount of non-reusable waste. However, many initiatives are on-going to increase the sustainability of research and reduce our carbon footprint where we can. At the LMS, one of the recent improvements we have made is to switch all paper products to recycled alternatives. This picture of the world is printed on recycled paper as a picture of health requires not only healthy people but a healthy planet, a concept which is in the palm of our hands to reach. Initiatives like these involve small steps which when applied to the entire institute can amount to a much larger change.

Greening LMS is a group of staff and student volunteers, working to improve sustainability at the institute. They have orchestrated many projects to improve and implement green, environmentally-friendly practices for scientific research as well as raising awareness for the impact of science on the environment and how this can be reduced. This photograph was taken by Julia Needham, a student member of the group, who oversaw the recycled paper project.

Elizabeth Cottier-Cook

MARINE BIOLOGIST

Elizabeth Cottier-Cook is Professor in Marine Biology, specialising in Marine Invasive Species and Biosecurity, at the Scottish Association for Marine Science and a Fellow of the Royal Society of Biology. She currently leads the GlobalSeaweedSTAR programme, a major international initiative funded by UKRI.

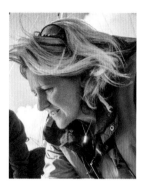

Millions of farmers, particularly women and their families, produce seaweed as a crop. This is used to produce food, cosmetics and ingredients used in everyday items on supermarket shelves worldwide, such as ice-cream, toothpaste and beer! Seaweeds require no additional fertilisers or freshwater, unlike terrestrial crops like wheat, and can grow 30 times faster than trees. Seaweeds can help us to tackle some of the biggest challenges our oceans face. Seaweeds help combat climate change by storing up carbon and moving it into the deep sea, where it can be locked away for centuries. They can also increase biodiversity by over 40% in areas where they are grown. Seaweeds are remarkable, however, entire crops can be lost to outbreaks of disease and pests, which are being made worse by climate change. Our work on the GlobalSeaweedSTAR project, led by the Scottish Association for Marine Science (SAMS) with partners across the world, is helping to identify these diseases and pests, to detect them earlier and to limit their spread. In this way, action can be taken before the whole crop is lost. We are also discovering more resilient seaweed varieties and looking for ways to improve the lives of seaweed farmers and the health of the environment that supports them.

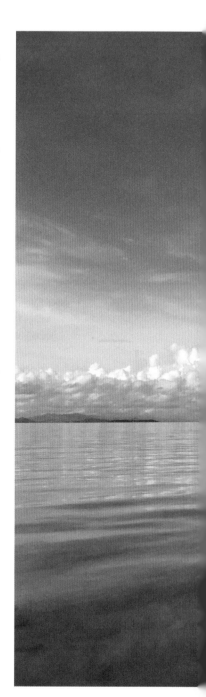

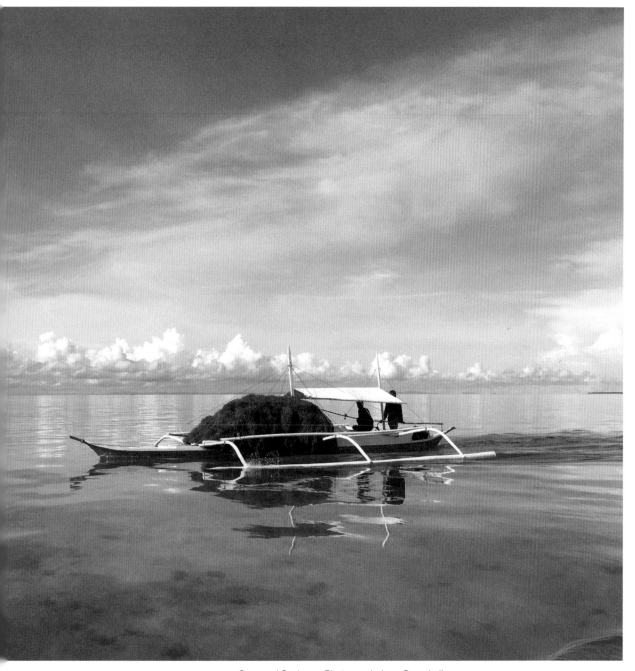

Seaweed Saviours. Photograph: Iona Campbell

Kyne Uhlig and Nikolaus Hillebrand
ANIMATORS FILM MAKERS

We all know that vegetables are important for a healthy diet but we still don't think enough about how they make their way to our tables. Instead of travelling huge distances, being stuck in traffic jams and arriving in CO_2 emitting trucks at our nearest supermarkets, shouldn't they use public transport and arrive by cargo bike directly at our doorstep?

When we spotted these vegetables waiting at a bus stop surrounded by thriving carrot and cabbage fields in the Garzweiler lignite mining area near Aachen we thought they were the best advertisement to make regional transport more attractive.

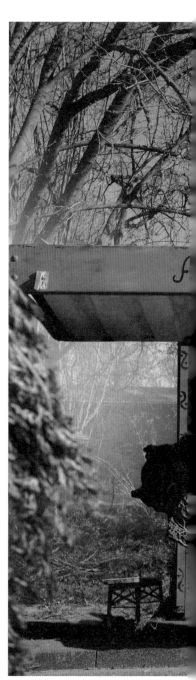

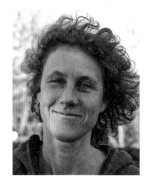

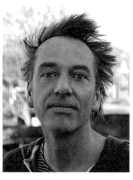

Kyne Uhlig and Nikolaus Hillebrand produce and create animated films for German TV, especially children's programs, as well as for independent films and music videos. Many of their films are also developed during participatory workshops they organise for local communities with a focus on environmental and musical education. They also teach animated film at the Cologne University of Applied Sciences.

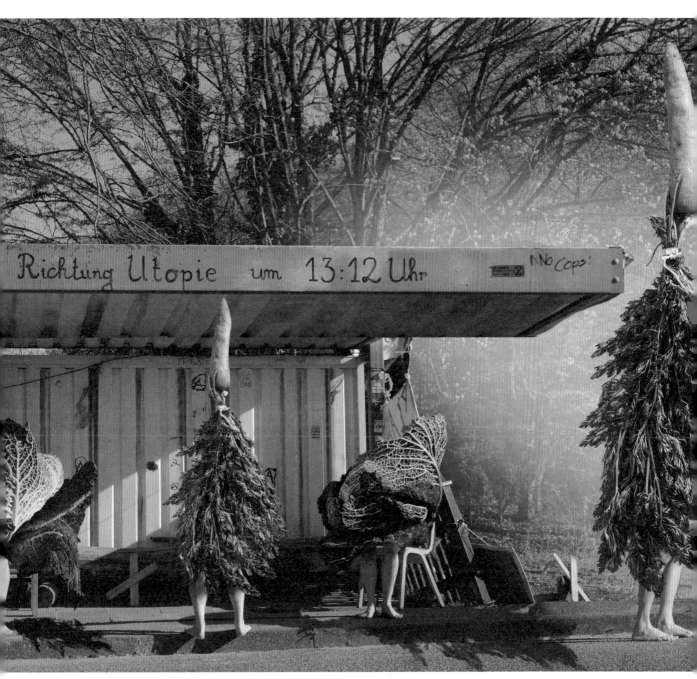

First Stop: Utopia at 13:12

James Frederick Barrett
VISUAL COMMUNICATOR

Cities are unhealthy places because they are completely artificial. They are false environments because they are out of touch with their origins in nature, they are nature after heavy processing from our imaginations. It is universally accepted that what is natural is healthy: a thing looks better when it is not contrived, a thing looks better when it is balanced and true to itself.

What comes to mind with *A Picture of Health* are images that are about how we balance out the city, and our interior environments with tokens of the natural world, flowers, house plants, gardens, parks – the place of the natural world in this way is about maintaining health, clarity, sanity in the midst of what is otherwise an entirely man-made environment. We'd get really lost without using nature in this way. Plants remind us where we've come from and what we knew for thousands of years. Any encounter with nature has the ability to stabilise us in our true heritage. We all came from nature, and we do our best in chaotic urban environments to remind ourselves and find relief in this, because the natural world is simpler and more honest than ours. So these images of plants are evidence of our attempts to maintain our health through this kind of balancing act.

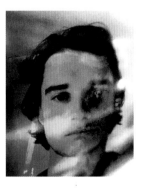

I graduated in 2018 from the University of East Anglia studying American Literature and Creative Writing and have been working as a photographer since, though I've been pursuing communication through visual arts from a much younger age. All my interests converge on expression through but not limited to visual means, making films, music, drawing... I'm at my best when trying to communicate abstraction.

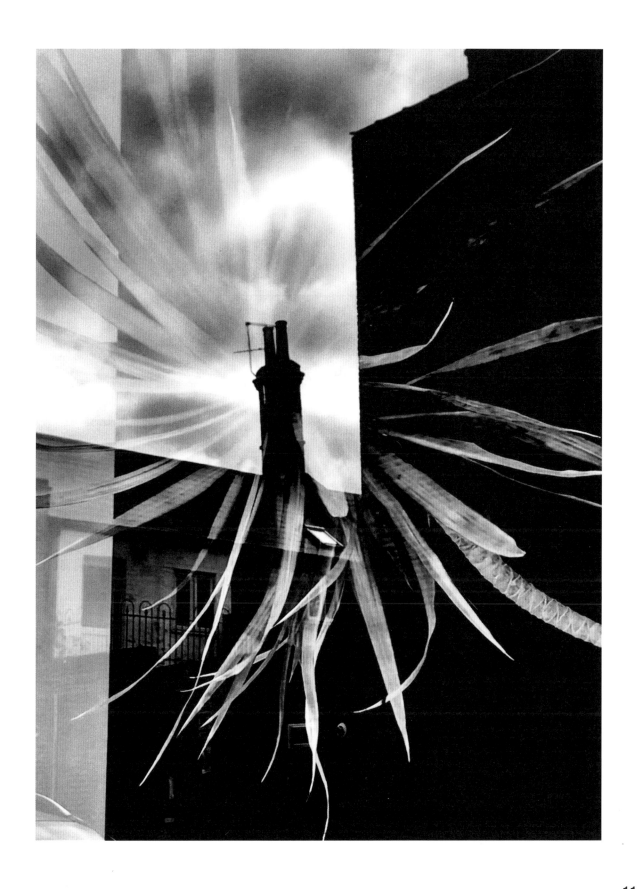

Ben Okri

POET NOVELIST PLAYWRIGHT

Ben Okri is a poet, novelist, and playwright. His novel The Famished Road *won the Booker Prize in 1991. His book* Astonishing the Gods *was chosen by the BBC as one of the most influential novels written over the last 300 years. He was born in Nigeria and lives in London. Recent work includes the novel* The Freedom Artist; *a volume of short stories* A Prayer for the Living; *and a new collection of poems* A Fire in my Head. *His latest book* Every Leaf a Hallelujah *is an environmental fairy tale for children and adults.*

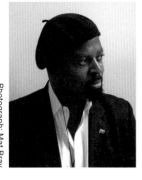

Photograph: Mat Bray

He was surprised to know, in a flash, without being told, that banks were places where people deposited or withdrew thoughts of well-being, thoughts of wealth, thoughts of serenity. When people were ill they went to their banks. When healthy, they went to the hospitals.

The hospitals were places of laughter, amusement, and recreation. They were houses of joy. The doctors and nurses were masters of the art of humour, and they all had to be artists of one kind or another.

It was a unique feature of the place, but the hospitals had their facades painted by the great masters of art. They were some of the most beautiful and harmonious buildings in the city. Merely looking at them lifted the spirits.

The masters of the land believed that sickness should be cured before it became sickness. The healthy were therefore presumed sick. Healing was always needed, and was considered a necessary part of daily life. Healing was always accompanied by the gentlest music. When healing was required the sick ones lingered in the presence of great paintings, and sat in wards where masterpieces of healing composition played just below the level of hearing. Outdoor activity, sculpting, story-telling, poetry, and laughter were the most preferred forms of treatment. Contemplation of the sea and of the people's origins and of their destiny was considered the greatest cure for sickness before it became sickness.

The inhabitants of that land, who were the hardest workers in the universe, were seldom ill. When they were ill at all, it was in order to regenerate their dreams and visions.

They went to the hospitals to improve their art of breathing. They went for stillness. They went there to remember their beginnings and to keep in mind their ever-elusive destination. Hospitals were places where the laws of the universe were applied. Individuals, mostly, healed themselves. The art of self-healing was the fourth most important aspect of their education.

Chapter 9 from Book 3 of Ben Okri's novel *Astonishing the Gods*

Hugo Williams

POET

The Deal

If you feel like a change
you can swap your present condition
for a case of dizziness,
bed for breathlessness,
cramps for unconsciousness.
You can lower your blood pressure
in return for a sick headache,
bore yourself to death
watching wheels going round,
or die of blood poisoning.

When you've cut some sort of deal
with the laws of nature
and passed another day on your back,
you can totter out of there
in thrall to the velvet hour,
sensing around you
the promise of night-scented streets
and the recklessness of summer.
You wonder what you would give
In exchange for this.

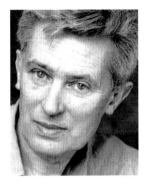

Hugo Williams was born in 1942 and grew up in Sussex. He worked on the London Magazine *from 1961 to 1970, since when he has earned his living as a journalist and travel writer.* Billy's Rain *won the T.S. Eliot Prize in 1999. His* Collected Poems *was published in 2002, and his last collection,* I Knew the Bride, *was published in 2014 and shortlisted for the Forward and the T.S. Eliot prizes. In 2004 he received the Queen's Gold Medal for Poetry.*

Alan Forsyth

ARCHITECT

All three images reflect a shared belief that Architecture can improve the human condition through the creation of places and environments that promote health and well-being in the broadest meaning of the words.

They may be seen to reflect the time and the place in which they were created, however all three convey a timeless message of hope and of optimism that is both irresistible and uplifting.

As we look to the future, they act as a reminder of the benefit of looking to the past in order to ensure that enduring truths and values may be learned afresh, re-imagined and given new life.

They demonstrate what can be achieved when there is a unity of purpose and vision.

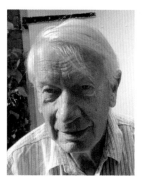

Born in Newcastle-upon-Tyne in 1944, Alan Forsyth remains a fervent Newcastle United supporter. He studied at The Architectural Association School of Architecture where he met and became friends with Gordon Benson. Together they worked for the London Borough of Camden Architects Department, from 1969–1978 being responsible for several innovative housing projects. In 1978 the practice of Benson & Forsyth Architects was formed. Their best-known built work includes the Museum of Scotland and the Millennium Wing of the National Gallery of Ireland.

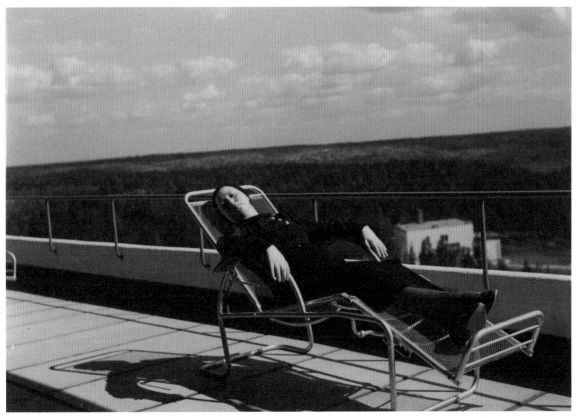

An outdoor terrace for patients in a Sanatorium situated in pine forests outside the town of Paimio in South Western Finland. Alvar Aalto 1929–1933. Courtesy of the Alvar Aalto Foundation, Finland

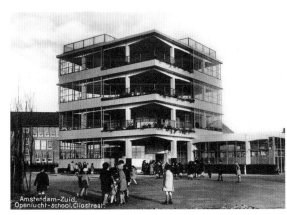

An Open Air School located within a residential court-yard in Central Amsterdam.
Jan Duiker 1927–1930. Courtesy of the Open Air School, Amsterdam

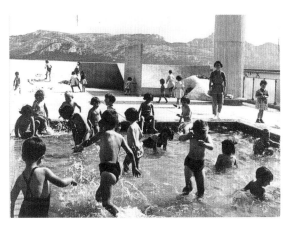

A kindergarten situated on a residential roof terrace located between the Sainte-Baume Mountains and the Mediterranean Sea.
Le Corbusier 1947–1952. Photograph: Louis SCIARLI (Archives municipales de Marseille, 47 Fi). © F.L.C. / ADAGP, Paris and DACS, London 2021

Chris Bowlby

JOURNALIST

For one extraordinary day in September, Tyneside goes running. Fifty-seven thousand this year, from elite athletes to every kind of age and ability, race, jog or amble their way on a half marathon from Newcastle's city centre.

First run in 1981, as the North East faced huge social and economic disruption, it has grown ever since. And those surging across the Tyne Bridge this autumn were celebrating the event's return after last year's loss to COVID-19.

Celebration is always the mood, amidst all the physical effort. Locals cheer, bands play, smiles are exchanged as a wave of mobile colour passes by. There is every kind of costume, and all sorts of kit advertising sponsorship for medical charities.

In a place still facing some of Britain's greatest health challenges, this is a day of joyful defiance, an annual running rebuke to the image of regional depression and hopeless decline.

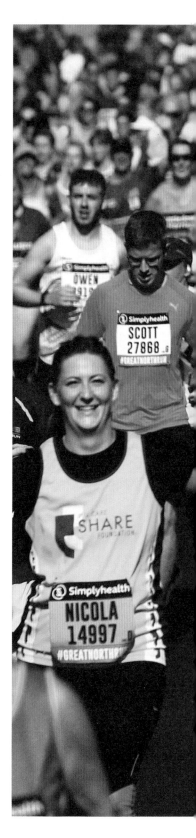

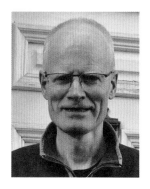

Chris Bowlby is a freelance writer and broadcaster based in North East England. He was for several decades a staff presenter and producer for BBC Radio, and was BBC Prague correspondent. He has written regularly for The Times *newspaper and the* BBC History *magazine.*

Born in Stockton on Tees he has also lived in the US and Germany. He ran the Great North Run for the first time in 1988, and then again in 2021.

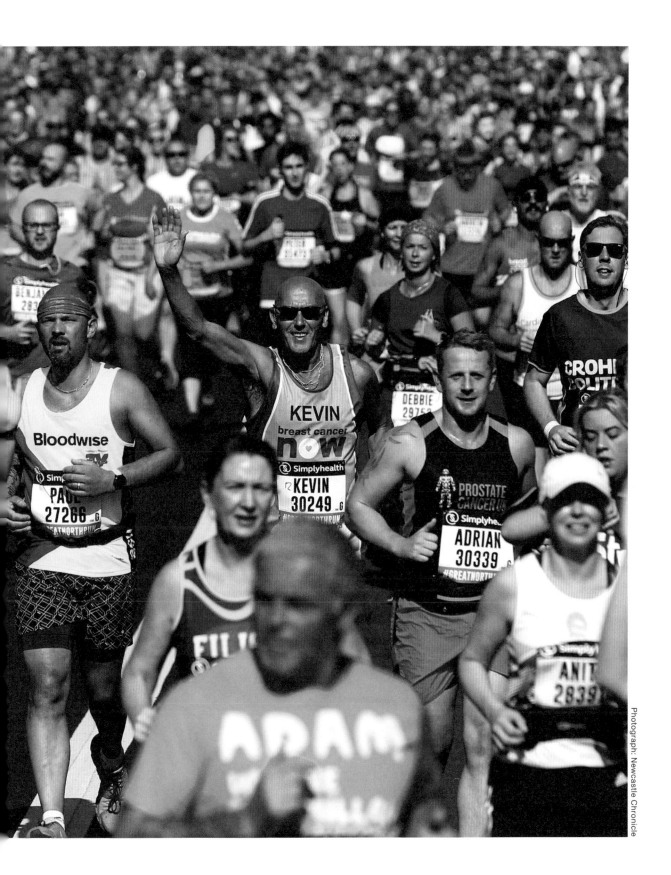

Photograph: Newcastle Chronicle

Sadiq Khan
MAYOR OF LONDON

London is the greatest city in the world, and the reason for that is you – the people who live here and keep our city's giant heart beating.

The last two years have been very difficult for us all as we've missed out on seeing friends or family, visiting our favourite venues, doing the things we love, and making the most of everything our wonderful city has to offer.

That's why my picture of health is seeing our city back where it belongs – our world-famous cultural heritage and attractions thriving, our businesses bouncing back and our city shining as a beacon for inclusion, a global hub for innovation and a creative hotbed that's overflowing with energy, ideas and imagination, where all Londoners have the opportunities to thrive.

We are roaring back as a city and working together to build the fairer, greener, safer and more prosperous capital all Londoners want and deserve.

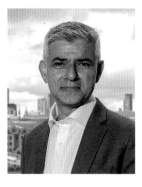

Sadiq Khan's parents moved from Pakistan to London in the 1960s, where he was born and has lived all his life. State-school educated in Tooting before studying Law at the University of North London, Sadiq became a solicitor specialising in human rights and was a London Borough of Wandsworth councillor from 1994–2006. Elected MP for Tooting in 2005, as Minister of State for Transport, he became the first Muslim and first Asian to attend Cabinet. In 2016 he was elected Mayor of London. Sadiq is a big sports fan and ran the 2014 London Marathon, raising money for the Evening Standard's Dispossessed Fund.

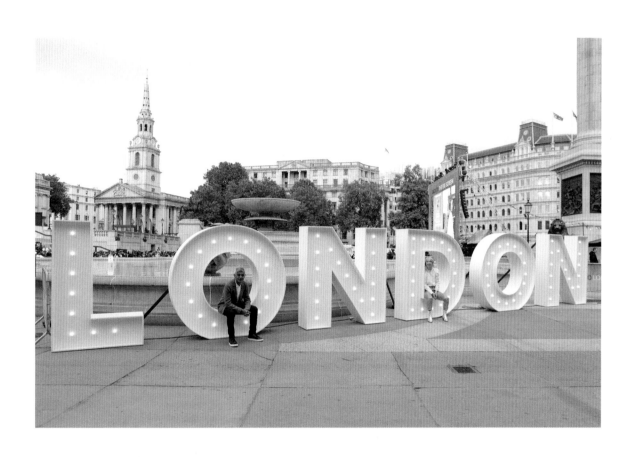

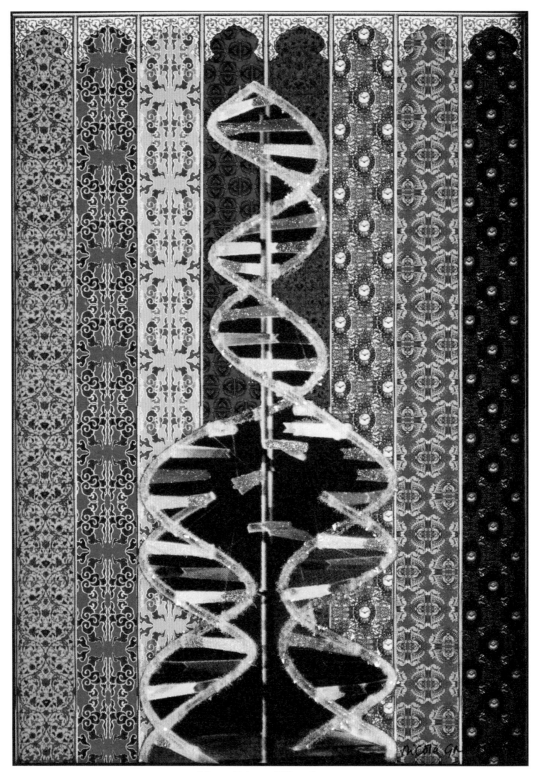

Advent, Major and Minor Groove
Gilding and painting on giclée, with hand applied diamond dust on 308gsm Hahnemuhle.
Dimensions H52 x W40 cm. © Nicola Green 2021

124

Nicola Green
ARTIST AND SOCIAL HISTORIAN

The two-stranded double helix structure of a DNA molecule is instantly recognisable as an iconic symbol of one of the most important scientific breakthroughs in human history. The discovery of disease-causing protein-coding genes represents a major shift in medicine from treating the symptoms of disease to treating the source.

I wanted to artistically render the flowing, almost arabesque, anti-parallel lines of the double helix whilst still portraying the intertwining corkscrew of the major and minor grooves as precisely and accurately as possible. This artwork depicts the replication of DNA from one double helix into two, the process that makes every cell in all living organisms; it is a component from which all human beings are made. DNA represents the story of humanity with a common genetic ancestry in Sub-Saharan Africa as well as carrying the genetic information that makes each of us unique. I sought to capture this in the bespoke patterned background which incorporates symbolically rich imagery drawn from different traditions around the world, all standing side-by-side behind the double helix structure.

I hope this artwork reflects how modern medicine has been inherently shaped by the transmission of knowledge, shared heritage, and cultural exchange; particularly the influence of traditional medicine from India, China and the Middle East. In doing so, this piece also represents the collaborative approach of the LMS to the advancement of human health and the diversity of London, one of the most multicultural cities in the world.

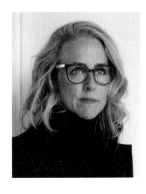

Nicola Green is a critically acclaimed artist and social historian. She has established an international reputation for her ambitious projects that can change perceptions about identity and power; exploring themes of inclusion, leadership, race and gender. She has gained unprecedented access to iconic figures from the worlds of religion, politics, and culture, including collaborations with Pope Francis, President Obama and the Dalai Lama. Driven by her belief in the power of the visual image to communicate important human stories, Nicola chooses to assume the role of 'witness' to momentous occasions taking place across the globe to create and preserve social-cultural heritage for future generations.

Avrn Justice
SHIP BREAKING WORKER

The photo was taken of Abu Nur Mia, 19 days before he passed away. He was born on 5 November, 1977 and died on 15 August 2020. It was the first time he got the chance to go to hospital since he was first diagnosed as an asbestos victim in 2017.

The workers were unaware of the harmful effects of asbestos in the ship breaking sector. The ship breaking yard owners in Bangladesh did not provide them scientific information. As a result, many workers were silently attacked by asbestos in the workplace. In 2017, the health survey by NGO the Bangladesh Occupational Safety, Health and Environment Foundation revealed the ship breaking workers' asbestos disaster. A health check of 100 workers identified 33 asbestos victims. Four of the 33 died without treatment. Many are on the verge of death due to serious illness, forced to live inhumane lives. Ship breaking owners, the government and international shipping organisations have not come forward to compensate and provide medical assistance to the workers. We think this is a crime against humanity. In the political reality of Bangladesh, the victims are not able to file a case in court. They deserve healthcare, justice and security.

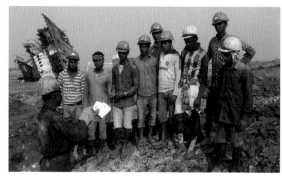

Avrn Justice providing informal information on asbestos at work

Avrn Justice*, born in 1971 in Bangladesh, started work in ship breaking aged 15. When the new labour law was passed in 2006 by parliament in Bangladesh he studied it and optimistically engaged in its implementation in the life of his fellow workers.

Soon the situation deteriorated. It became harder and harder to receive the £1,000 compensation for fully invalided workers. In 2017 he tested positive for asbestosis – like 32 others among the 100 long term ship breaking workers.
*Not his real name.

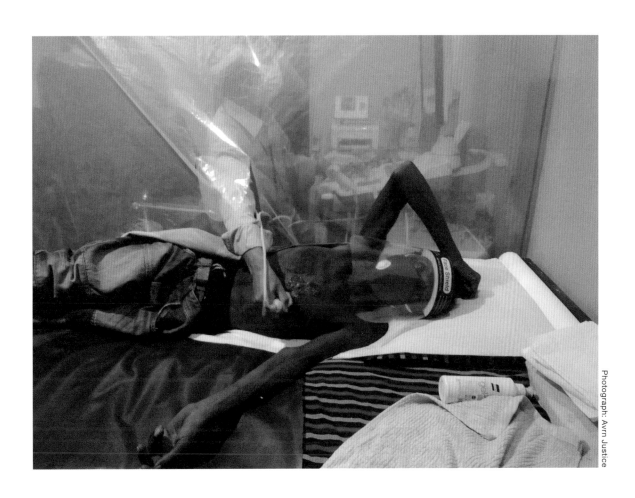

Anukta
SHIP BREAKING WORKER

At the beginning when I started working in ship breaking aged 17 I kind of liked it working on the big vessels high above the forests and the sea. Only later I found out it was all bad. Ship breaking is a hazardous industry. An average of 20 workers die each year, and many are paralyzed in accidents.

Workers work with serious health risks. They do not have adequate safety equipment. A cutting operator is exposed to toxic fumes for an average of 8 hours daily. Most of the workers here work for 25 to 30 years and suffer from severe diseases, such as cancer and asbestosis, and head, eye, ear and skin problems.

Workers are not adequately trained about toxins or asbestos. They have to work hard for about 11 hours, 6 days a week. Every day the workers get sick when they return home. There is no economic security, social security, or job security. We feel that ship breaking owners, international ship owners, and shipping company owners are all responsible for this exploitation in the ship breaking industry.

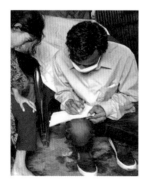

Anukta taking interviews for a food program during the COVID-19 pandemic

Anukta*, born 1982 in Bangladesh, started ship breaking aged 17. For more than a decade he has been striving to raise awareness of hazardous materials at work and for labour rights among the ship breaking workers. He makes sure his voice is heard by the yard owners and, when accidents occur, by the government agency for health and safety inspection. It is a risky life.
*Not his real name

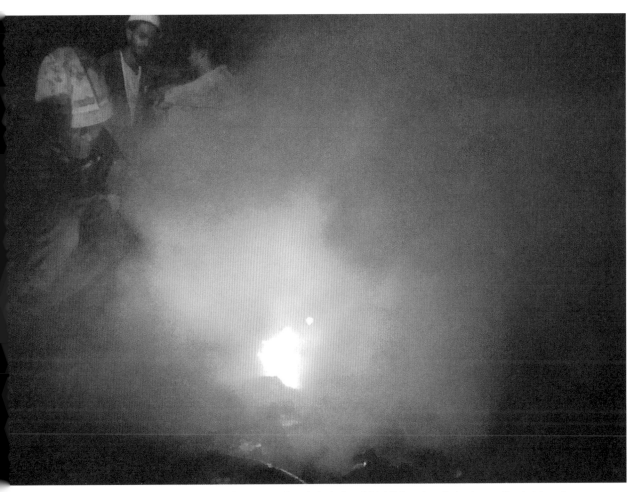

Cutterman ship breaking in Chittagong, Bangladesh; the nightshift is not carried out according to labour law. Smoke from dry waste oil on the ship walls mixes with steam. Photographs: Avrn Justice

Kevin Fenton

PUBLIC HEALTH REGIONAL DIRECTOR

I have always been drawn to sunsets. Perfect sunsets. Ones where the sun takes its time to meander towards and beyond the vast horizon, changing its colour, warmth, and intensity. Growing up in the Caribbean, my earliest memories were of red-golden perfect sunsets, the taste of warm ocean breeze, the laughter of family and friends accompanied by relentless, rhythmic crashing waves. These were my earliest lessons in connecting with others, learning to appreciate the beauty and power of nature. Today, perfect sunsets remain an important part of my life, invoking feelings of closure, stillness, and gratitude. They gift me time to pause and reflect on my wellbeing – how I think and feel, my satisfaction with life, my blessings and challenges, meaning and purpose. They remind me that health truly is more than the absence of disease or infirmity, but a state of complete physical, mental, social and spiritual wellbeing.

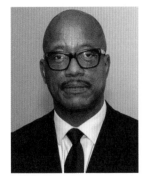

Professor Kevin Fenton is a senior public health expert and infectious disease epidemiologist, who has worked in a variety of public health executive leadership roles across government and academia in the UK and internationally, including taking a leading role in London's response to the COVID-19 pandemic. Currently Regional Director for Public Health, Office for Health Improvement and Disparities and Statutory Health Advisor to the Mayor of London, Greater London Authority and London Assembly, he has recently been elected as the next President of the UK Faculty of Public Health. In 2022, he was awarded a CBE for services to public health.

Francis Crick Institute
BIOMEDICAL RESEARCH INSTITUTE

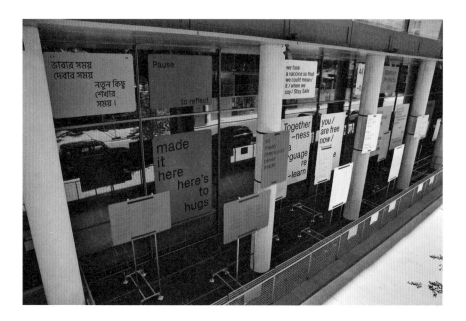

Now, more than ever, we are appreciating the impact that science has on our everyday lives. The Crick's pop-up poetry exhibition, *A Drop of Hope*, was inspired by the words of those who received a COVID-19 vaccine at the Francis Crick Institute, the reflections of our volunteers, and the experiences of our local communities. Written by twelve virtual poets in residence, the project celebrated the individual contribution of each vaccine recipient to the wider community and global scientific effort.

Nazneen is a writer, historian and creative writing facilitator.

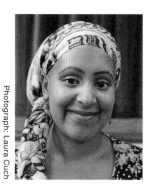

Photograph: Laura Cuch

Reflecting the growing participation in the vaccine programme, the installation was installed in three phases. The poems created a rainbow-like form, a symbol that became synonymous with hope during the COVID-19 pandemic. Nazneen Ahmed's poem 'Dhonnobad' is just one of the twelve poems written in English, Bengali and Somali, available to read or listen to on the Crick's website.

'Dhonnobad' by Nazneen Ahmed

ধন্যবাদ

The word 'dhonnobad' in Bangla
Is near-to untranslateable
The closest to a meaning in English might
    be 'I acknowledge your goodness
and speak my blessings upon you.'

As I sit with the life fluttering within me
Afraid for us both and helpless
I am calm too in this knowing
That each of you will keep us safe.
That means more than I have
    English words to say.

So

To each of you standing in the queue,
Waiting for the shot in your arm,
From me and my unborn child:
ধন্যবাদ

To each of you who have walked past here
On your precious hour of calm,
From me and my unborn child:
ধন্যবাদ

To each of you within these walls
Gentling the afraid, your kindness a balm
From me and my unborn child:
ধন্যবাদ

To each of you within the labs
Searching for ways to keep us from harm
From me and my unborn child:
ধন্যবাদ

To each of you who made the
    hardest choices
Setting aside your qualms
From me and my unborn child:
ধন্যবাদ

To each of you
Placing a drop of hope
Into this bitter ocean of fear and pain
It is your
        single
            drop
That will turn it sweetly salt again

And me and my unborn child
Reach out from our hearts with this refrain:
ধন্যবাদ.

It means the world.

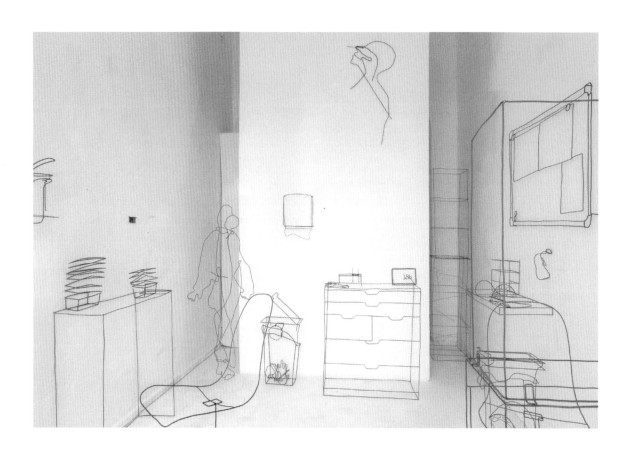

Sibylle Hofter
VISUAL ARTIST

The installation is a spatial drawing of a coronavirus test centre, made for and showcased at the project space Berlin-Weekly. In the installation, one moves through a space in which furnishings and utensils typical of coronavirus test centres are sketched out of welded wire just enough for the eye to see surfaces where there are none. The movement of the viewer shifts the perspective to the spatial relationships, in which the back edges of the objects are always visible.

The cityscape characterized by COVID-19 (with empty streets, faces hidden behind masks and closed shops and restaurants) and the shop spaces converted into test centres have become part of everyday life for most of us during the many months of the lockdown, but the unique phenomenon of the test centre seems to have been documented surprisingly little artistically.

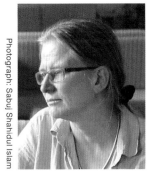

Photograph: Sabuj Shahidul Islam

Sibylle Hofter is a Berlin-based visual artist exploring film, text, site-specific sculpture, installation in public space and primarily photography. She is also a curator of various projects, and initiator of diverse Büro Schwimmer long term projects. Her working process usually includes extensive research on extra-cultural fields. Currently she focuses on emancipatory, post-colonial, collaborative processes – being art or beyond.

Ian Pollock

ILLUSTRATOR

In the early months of the lockdown these hunched, hooded and masked creatures emerged from behind the urban wainscoting onto the otherwise deserted streets, each pushing a dog on a string as if, with a metal detector, scanning along a strandline of discarded surgical masks.

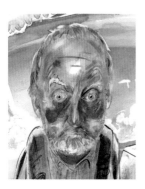

Born in 1950, Ian Pollock studied at Manchester College of Art and Design then moved to London to gain an MA at the Royal College of Art. He spent the next 20 years in London working as an illustrator for most of the major newspapers, supplements and magazines on both sides of the Atlantic including The Times, Observer, New Yorker, Penthouse, Playboy and Rolling Stone. In the late 90's he returned to his roots in Cheshire continuing to work as an illustrator. He was awarded an Honorary Degree of Doctor of Arts, Wolverhampton University in 2001.

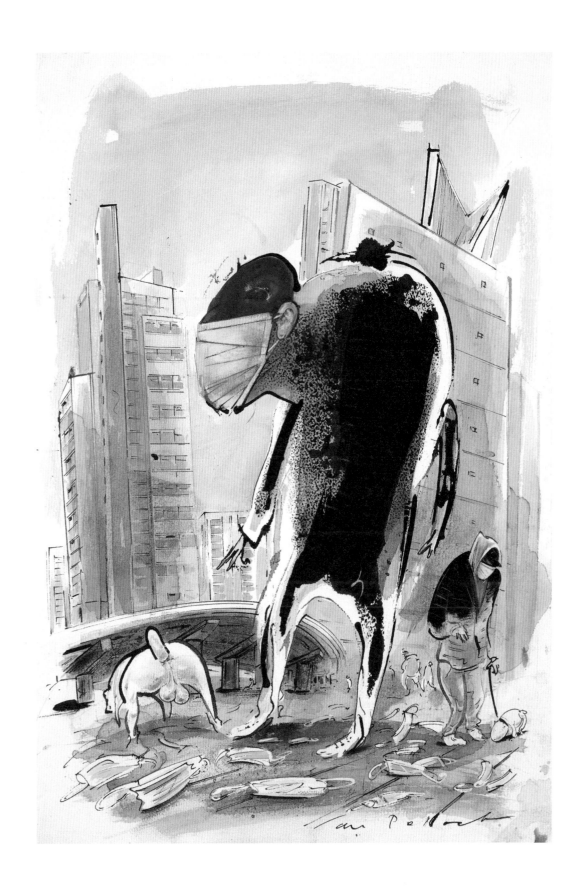

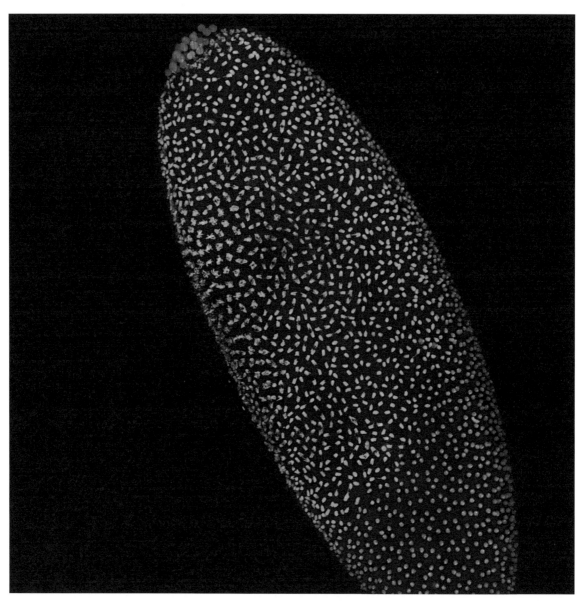

And a new life awakens. Photograph: Liz Ing-Simmons

Juanma Vaquerizas

GENOME BIOLOGIST

Animals of all kinds must go through zygotic genome activation: After fertilisation the first developmental steps are enabled from the maternally inherited material. Then a switch occurs to full control of the developmental programme which will form a new individual using their own genome.

Here this transition is happening in a fruit fly embryo. We can see the majority of nuclei in the embryo undergoing nuclear division (in blue), with a special compartment of cells called pole cells (pink) that will lead to the formation of the germline.

Zygotic genome activation represents fundamental aspects in the life of all animal species, including ourselves. It represents the success of a whole developmental programme for the parents, and for the species as a whole, in which the genetic information of a species is encapsulated into gametes and passed to the next generation. It represents a challenge for the new organism, where its genome must ensure that starting from the blank canvas of a single cell – the zygote – a plethora of cell types and functions are deployed in a timely fashion to produce a fully formed new individual. Finally, it represents evolution, since the very same mechanisms that lead to the generation of the enormous cellular complexity of an organism will also lead to mutations that can be incorporated and fixed in the genome of the species driving their evolution.

Zygotic genome activation is an amazing time point in the life of any organism, one that we should carefully study and marvel at how nature managed to orchestrate it.

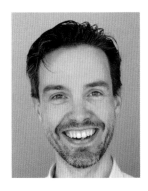

Professor Juanma Vaquerizas has been an MRC Investigator and Programme Leader at the LMS since 2019, and is Chair in Developmental and Regulatory Genomics at Imperial College London. His main research contributions include the discovery of the timing and molecular mechanisms involved in the establishment of the three-dimensional organisation of the genome during early embryonic development. Juanma received his PhD from the Spanish National Cancer Centre and Universidad Autónoma de Madrid, Spain. After postdoctoral training with Nick Luscombe at EMBL–European Bioinformatics Institute in Cambridge, UK he was awarded a Max Planck Research Group at MPI-Muenster, Germany.

James Le Fanu
GP AND WRITER

The long march in pursuit of a cure for childhood acute lymphocytic leukaemia ranks amongst the most impressive of all medical achievements, vividly portrayed in this graph published in the journal *Blood* in 1971, just over fifty years ago. The challenge could not have been more formidable, predicated on the separate discovery of five novel anti-cancer drugs each working in a radically different way. Then it was necessary to establish a vast intellectual machine of clinical trials to assess the outcome of various treatment combinations. Finally, the patients were children and the drugs very toxic. It needed an extraordinary sense of purpose to persist when many doctors thought it immoral to subject children to their cruel side effects for the minimal gain of postponing, often for only a few months, death from a lethal illness.

The breakthrough only came with the brave decision by Dr Donald Pinkel of St Jude's Hospital in Memphis to intensify treatment yet further, doubling the dose of radiotherapy to the brain and administering the cytotoxic drug methotrexate directly into the spinal fluid – in anticipation of eliminating residual leukaemic cells in the central nervous system. The outcome, as revealed by the graph was dramatic. Whereas virtually all the children in previous cohorts eventually relapsed, with this new regime 70% were still in complete remission after three years. Yet further refinements and improvements in treatment over the next three decades would push the cure rate up to a previously unimaginable 91%. There was, noted *The Lancet,* "now no place for the palliative treatment of leukaemia."

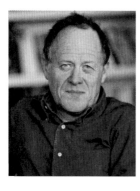

James Le Fanu is a doctor, columnist, social commentator and historian of science and medicine. He graduated from Cambridge University and the Royal London Hospital in 1974. He subsequently worked in the Renal Transplant Unit and Cardiology Departments of the Royal Free and St Mary's Hospital in London. For twenty years he has combined working in General Practice with writing a weekly column for the Daily Telegraph *as well as contributing reviews and articles to* The Times, Spectator, Prospect, The British Medical Journal *and* Journal of the Royal Society of Medicine. *His books include* The Rise and Fall of Modern Medicine *and* Too Many Pills.

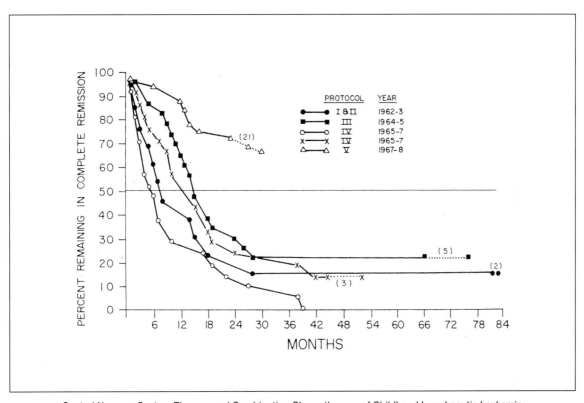

Central Nervous System Therapy and Combination Chemotherapy of Childhood Lymphocytic Leukemia
By Rhomes J.A. Aur, Joseph Simone, II. Omar Hunt, Thomas Walters, Luis Borella, Charles Pratt and Donald Pinkel.
Reproduced with permission from the American Society of Hematology.
Published in *Blood*, Vol. 37, No. 3 (March), 1971

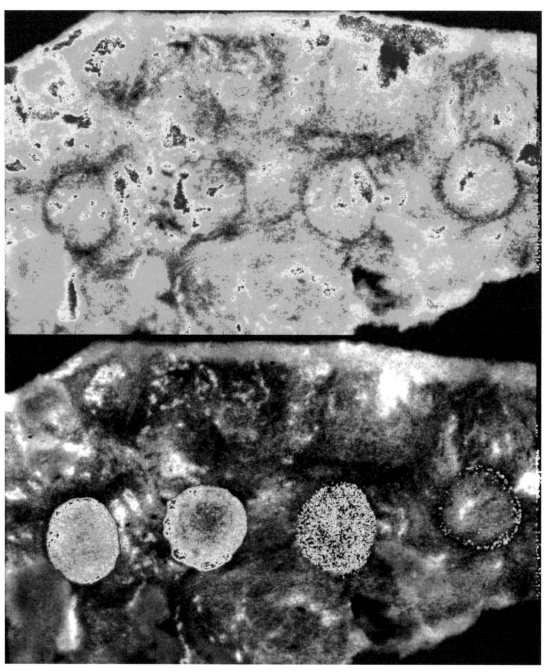

Image by Carmen Ramírez Moncayo, a second year PhD student in the Drug Transport and Tumour Metabolism lab

Louise Fets

CANCER BIOLOGIST

Over the last decade treatment options for cancer patients have improved dramatically, but with every therapy, there is patient-to-patient variability in treatment response. Of many potential factors that could play into this varied response, drug access to the tumour is an important one. Tumour vascularity has been widely studied, but how drugs enter cells is significantly less well understood.

We are trying to understand the role that proteins in cell membranes called transporters play in drug uptake. The level or 'expression' of these proteins varies significantly from one patient to another, and can even change between different regions of the same tumour. We believe that transporter expression patterns may be one of the factors that could predict response to therapy.

Mass spectrometry imaging (MSI) allows us to visualise the molecular architecture of a tissue, and we are developing MSI methods to see how drugs are distributed across a tumour. Our focus here is on a group of drugs called PARP inhibitors. These have been shown to significantly improve life expectancy for ovarian cancer patients. This picture shows how we have tested our methods on a sample of high-grade serous ovarian carcinoma tissue. The upper panel shows the distribution of a prevalent fatty molecule, highlighted by the spectrum of colours. Below, we have used the method to highlight four different PARP inhibitors applied as droplets onto the tissue. Our aim is to use this method on PARP inhibitor-dosed tissues to better understand what determines drug distribution within a tumour, with a long-term goal of being able to better predict which drugs a patient is likely to benefit from.

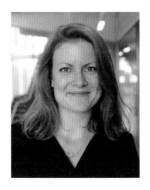

Louise is head of the Drug Transport and Tumour Metabolism lab, which opened in 2019 at the LMS. Louise completed a PhD at the MRC Laboratory of Molecular Biology, with a focus on cell motility and signal transduction before moving fields to study cancer metabolism during her postdoc at the Francis Crick Institute. Her current research aims to understand how transporter proteins mediate drug uptake, and how this intersects with their role in cancer metabolism.

Maithreyi Narasimha
CELL AND DEVELOPMENTAL BIOLOGIST

Tissue barriers – like the skin and the lining of the gut – that protect our exterior and interiors are essential for a healthy, working body, whether it's keeping the bad stuff out or the good stuff in. To probe the dynamics of how tissue barriers form during development we study fruit flies. This sequence of images from my lab shows the formation of a continuous epithelial barrier around the fly embryo by cell sheet migration and fusion. How this happens resembles not only how wounds heal but also how the palate and neural tube (the beginnings of the nervous system) are formed. By fluorescently tagging a protein called actin (dark stripes in the images) that powers cells to change shape and move, we watched in real time how the two flanks of the outer barrier – the skin of the fly – fuse to cover and protect the embryo. This showed us that cells (within each dark stripe) in the flanks of fusing sheets change in number and geometry to ensure that the edges of the stripes are precisely matched. Once fusion is complete the cells in the sheets interlock to form a strong and stable seal. Being able to see this at high resolution and in real time allows us to understand how genes and forces ensure the formation of healthy tissue barriers, and to obtain insights into the causation of epithelial diseases (including due to diabetes) that affect sheet integrity.

Well-designed architectural structures also rely on strong seals and barriers, so it seems very fitting that this image – as featured on the LMS's BPoD, called 'Fusing Fronts' and described by Lux Fatimathas – has inspired the pattern on the entrance facade of the new LMS research building.

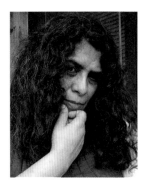

Maithreyi Narasimha is a Principal Investigator at the Department of Biological Sciences at the Tata Institute of Fundamental Research, Mumbai India. She studied medicine as an undergraduate in Bangalore, India and did her doctoral research on genomic imprinting with Prof. Azim Surani at the Gurdon Institute, University of Cambridge, UK. She was a postdoctoral fellow at the University of Cologne (with Prof. Maria Leptin) and at the University of Cambridge (with Prof. Nick Brown), where she developed her interest in understanding how epithelia are shaped. Her research broadly aims at understanding the molecular, cellular and physical bases of epithelial organisation and dynamics during development and disease.

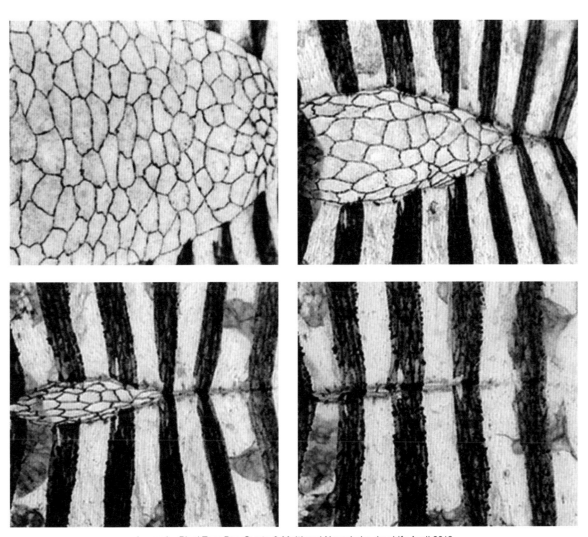

Image by Piyal Taru Das Gupta & Maithreyi Narasimha, in *eLife* April 2019

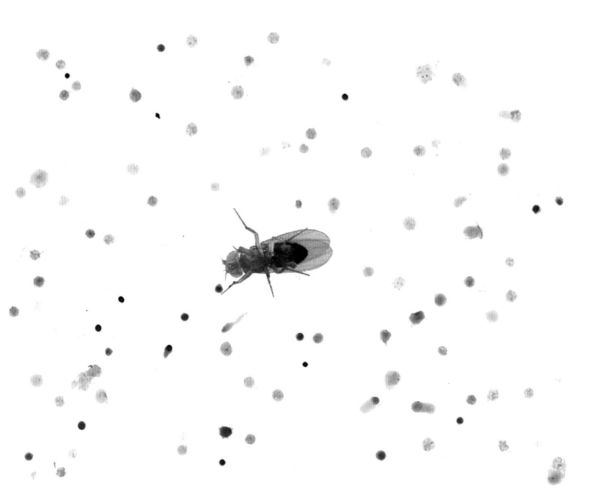

Dropping hints

Irene Miguel-Aliaga

BIOLOGIST

The fruit fly *Drosophila melanogaster* has been used for over 100 years to investigate how genes make an animal and what goes wrong as the animal ages or 'malfunctions'.

Over a decade ago, the first PhD student in my lab, Paola Cognigni, and myself had an idea: might we be able to use a fly's droppings to learn about what goes on inside it? This turned out to be a fruitful approach! It led us to many unexpected findings, some of which are relevant to us humans.

At the time, we joked about our flies having plagiarised Damien Hirst's spot paintings. We also fantasised about human health applications: could we invent toilet paper that would change colour to tell us about our sugar or cholesterol levels, or whether the right kind of microbes lived in our guts?

As is often the case, scientific creativity went beyond our wildest dreams, and I have been pleasantly surprised that testing wastewater for traces of viruses has helped tackle COVID-19 outbreaks.

Progress comes from unexpected places, and translating and applying fundamental discoveries to improve human health requires ingenuity and sometimes takes unexpected paths. It also needs a research environment that nurtures and supports both.

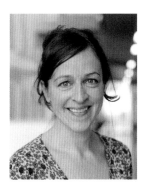

Irene Miguel-Aliaga is Professor of Genetics and Physiology at Imperial College London, and MRC Investigator at the LMS. Irene has an interest in the idiosyncrasies of adult organs: how and why they differ between males and females, and how they change depending on diet or internal state. Her lab has focused on the crosstalk between the brain and the gut to explore these questions. She spends her spare time nurturing the brains and the guts of two young children and a black and white cat.

Jerry Yi Chang

MEDICAL STUDENT

The future of medicine is a holistic one. Every patient should be seen and cared for as the diverse, individual 'whole', rather than as entities defined by their diagnoses. My picture of health illustrates this with a 'spectrum' of people varying in age, gender, ethnicity, and emotions, yet are still interconnected. While a healthcare professional's job requires clinical skill and knowledge, at its core it is always about people.

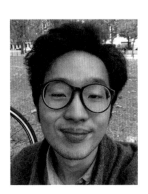

I am a final year medical student at King's College London, with also a Masters in Neuroscience. Having grown up in Taiwan, Australia, then the UK, I am endlessly drawn to the kaleidoscopic nature of people and minds. I explore this through pursuing psychiatry and creating art.

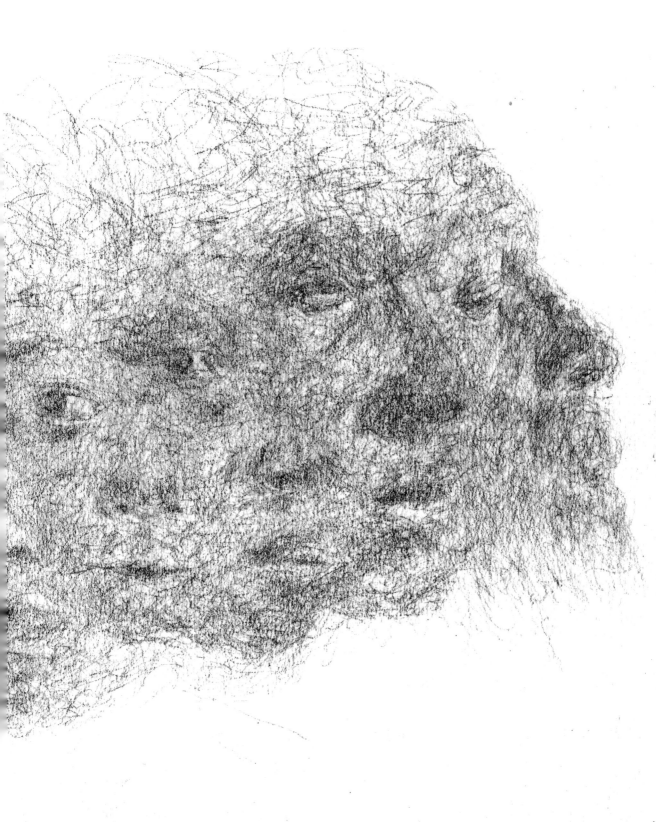

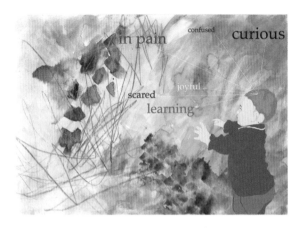

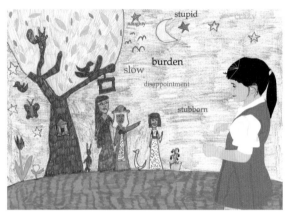

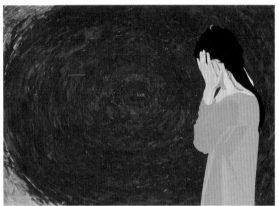

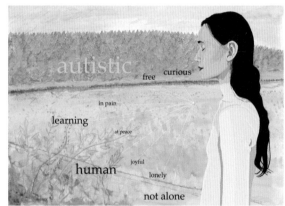

Dorota Ali and Francesca Happé

NEUROSCIENCE PhD STUDENT AND
COGNITIVE NEUROSCIENTIST

At different times and in different places, the phrase 'healthy autistic person' may sound like an oxymoron. More recently, however, disability rights movements, countless personal accounts, and many researchers and clinicians, have strongly emphasised that an autistic person is a whole, healthy, feeling and empathising human being.

With these images of transition – from toddlerhood to childhood to adolescence to adulthood – we wanted to capture changing perceptions of the self and of the world, drawing on both personal and wider stories. Transition reflects the interaction between innate differences (e.g., sensory, communication and language differences; high anxiety) and environmental factors that can cause real and chronic challenges (e.g., loud, fast-paced settings; lack of understanding; stigma). A diagnosis of autism can be a signpost on this journey to greater self-acceptance and should lead to more compassionate and equitable responses from others.

Above all, we wanted to highlight that, no matter the developmental course, no matter the diagnosis, every human being has a need to be understood, to be loved, and to be supported in their learning, growth, and – ultimately – health.

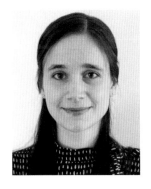

As an artist, I combine short stories and poetry with illustrations. I am also an Economic and Social Research Council-funded PhD student, learning about wellbeing and burnout in autistic populations. I draw on my personal experience, and a love for research and art.

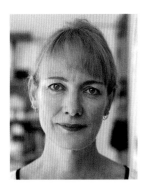

I am a psychologist who has spent 30 years trying to understand autism through a variety of methods, including working with experts-by-experience and artists.

Manon Ouimet

PHOTOGRAPHER

The body and its form are mostly seen as a disfiguration once you lose a part of your body... but this process really has helped me to embrace who I am. Another turning point on my road of self-discovery.

Tim, sitter from ALTERED

ALTERED is a body of photographic work that aims to encourage inclusion by displaying the honesty of physical alterations. It focuses on individuals who have unwillingly embarked on life-changing body alterations due to illness, war, accidents and violence. The intention is to illuminate people who often feel marginalised and contribute to conversations about equality and diversity. The work asks the viewer to explore themselves through the prism of others and to challenge or confirm their belief system regarding body image and its representation. The process of making these works also aims to encourage the sitters to increase their confidence and reclaim their identity, employing the practice of the 'therapeutic gaze' whereby the artistic process can take its participants on an emotional journey of self-discovery.

ALTERED was born from wanting to learn people's stories and champion the beauty of each individual.

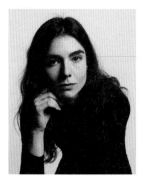

I started out taking portraits, quickly realising that for me photography is a vehicle with which to explore my relationship with what it means to be human, be it through others as the subject, or, occasionally, turning the camera onto myself. I got my MA at the University of the West of England where I made my award-winning project ALTERED, a series that focused on people who have been subject to life-altering bodily changes. My work explores the function and composition of the human form and I'm ever focusing on identity, visual representation and celebrating the body in abstracted and sculptural capacities.

Portrait of Damian

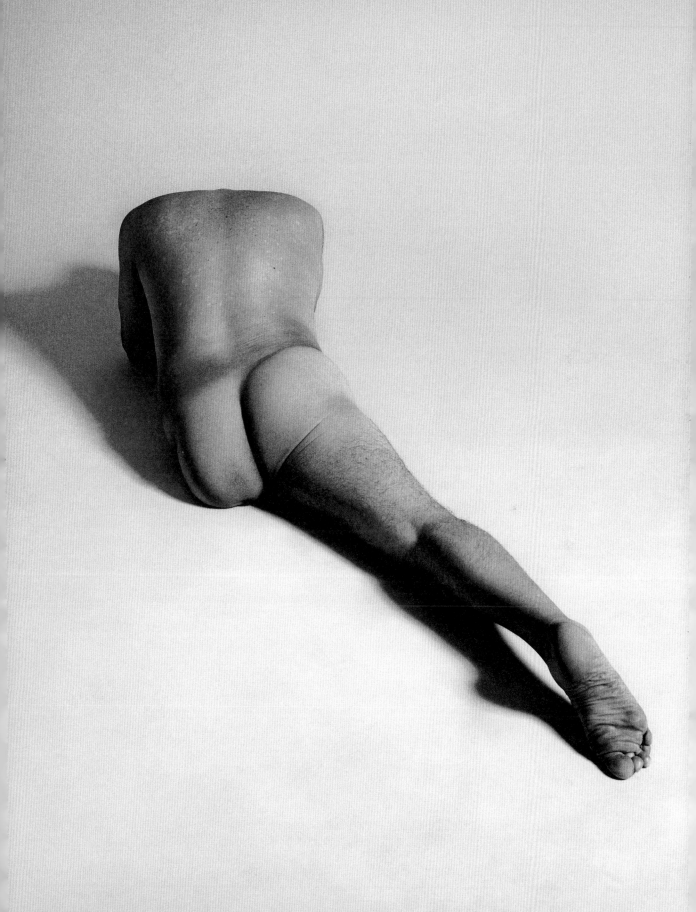

David Parker

PHOTOGRAPHER

Did this young man tip the Chevy into the 'levee', or did it somehow land there from outer space, all sci-fi blue with barely a scratch? That it might be an alien craft is not so far fetched; this is Nazca, where epic lines and animal geoglyphs etched into the desert by a lost civilisation have long spawned theories about ancient spacemen.

I was in Nazca working on a photo-book, *Broken Images*, and one aspect was the collision of belief systems – ancient, modern and scientific – in a place which had acquired cult status. I guess this picture shows that I too was susceptible to seeing things in terms of the pseudo-liminal zone that was Nazca.

This young sun-bronzed Heracles with enigmatic smile and mantle casually thrown over his shoulder, the very picture of vigorous physical good health, has the look of someone who knows something we don't. "I failed to ask him, 'Is this a drunken accident or a land art installation?'"

On a return visit to Nazca the following year I showed the picture to a friend who lived there. "Pity you weren't around a month later ... same car, different ditch!" Astonished, I again neglected to ask the obvious question, but in retrospect am glad I didn't. As long as I remain ignorant of the circumstances I can still bathe in the mystery and play with different scenarios; for me a healthy state of mind too.

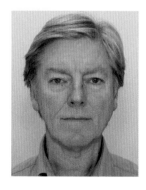

David Parker was born in Stafford, 1949, where he studied engineering and technical illustration before developing careers in commercial and scientific illustration and photography. He has produced three photographic monographs of personal work including Broken Images, *the award winning* The Phenomenal World, *and* Myth and Landscape. *The last two projects comprise large-format landscapes inspired by the pioneering 19th century topographic photographers. His work is represented by galleries in London, Hamburg and San Francisco.*

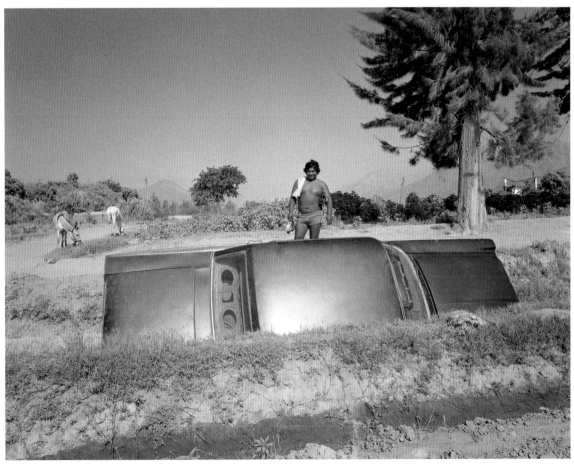

Irrigation Ditch with Taxi. Nazca, Peru 1988

...he should prefer not to know the sources of the Nile, and
that there should be some unknown regions preserved
as hunting-grounds for the poetic imagination.

GEORGE ELIOT

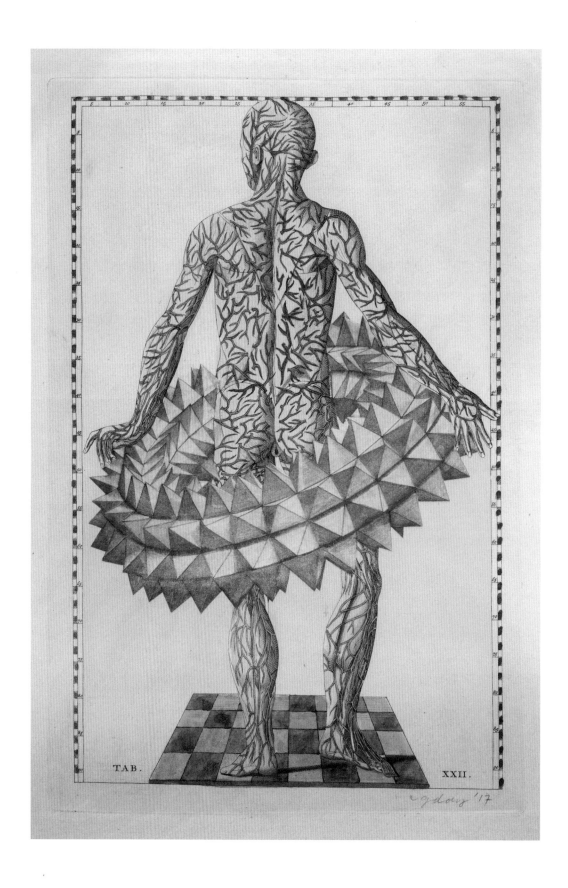

TAB.   XXII.

156

Graham Day

FINE ARTIST

I choose my collage (Blood Man) for *A Picture of Health* ironically because it looks distinctly unhealthy. I found the 17th century engraving of the bloody man in a flea market and wondered what it illustrated, something obviously caused all those punctures. My creative gene sought to suggest an answer and when I came across an illustration of a *mazzocchio* (part of a renaissance headgear) from Lorenzo Sirigatti's book *La Pratica di Prospettiva,* (Venice 1596) of a vicious looking device I wrapped it around the unfortunate bloody man to provide a possible explanation.

Unlike science, art mysteriously allows the viewer to provide their own unique interpretation of an image, as the greatest scientist of his age stated "The most beautiful thing we can experience is the mysterious. It is the source of all true art and science. He to whom the emotion is a stranger, who can no longer pause to wonder and stand wrapped in awe, is as good as dead — his eyes are closed".

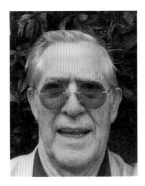

Born in London in 1946, Graham Day studied at Hornsey School of Art, Bath Academy of Art and University College London Slade School of Fine Art. He has been exhibiting in the UK and abroad since the early Seventies, and his work is part of prominent collections such as the British Museum, Victoria & Albert Museum, British Library, and the Bibliotheque Nationale in Paris.

Susan Mesinai

POET

War baby, mystic and grandmother – I was raised to honour not only science but prayer in healing. But the world taught me to put the spiritual last. The universal threat of the COVID-19 pandemic changed that. One night recently I looked up from my desk and gazed into the surrounding darkness. Rather than a Void I saw the Vastness of the Subtle, its rich essence and how invisibly it sustains all of us. Spice was written in that instant.

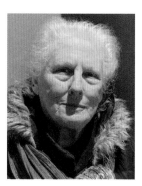

Poet and Columbia University graduate with High Honors in Comparative Religion, Susan Mesinai is best known for her human rights work in Russia to determine the fate of Raoul Wallenberg and other Disappeared.

I am Spice
With every incident of flesh
Each event, whether
In Time or Timelessness
Every breath –
A fragrance released to Memory

I weather the waves of Desire
To embrace the Subtle
A realm far more vast than
Excelsior could ever hope
to conquer.

Unlike the metals hewn

and perfected in dragon's fire
Then gold to dross again
I am Spice, wildflower petals
In a hamsin
The Infinity of a weedless
Garden where insects hum
But not as loud as the Spirits
In my room upon
Awakening

I am Spice in my well lit
Weightless Emptiness
I lay down my arms
Limbless, non violent in
Essence and yet
I embrace

Here in this endless Holy Space
Where Love attracts only
The Good
I am all and nothing
A scent, a
Barely visible presence.

I am Spice.

Jane Goodall, Giles Yeo and Clare Goodall

RESEARCH SCIENTIST, NEUROSCIENTIST AND STORYTELLER

A healthy neuronal circuitry between the different control centres of the brain involved in appetite and food intake is important to maintain a healthy body weight. There are, broadly speaking, three control regions. The fuel sensor, formed of the paraventricular (PVN) and arcuate (ARC) nuclei in the hypothalamus; the visceral centre in the hindbrain, which signals fullness and illness; and the reward centre, which makes eating feel nice. In this sculpture, the coloured lattice represents the overlapping layers of neuronal projections to these centres that occur in our brain.

From the fuel sensor in the hypothalamus, red threads represent neurons that stop eating (anorexigenic), green threads those increasing food intake (orexigenic). Yellow threads represent neurons projecting from the hindbrain to the reward centre signalling a spectrum from pleasant to unpleasant. Purple threads represent neurons projecting from the reward centre to the rest of the brain.

This textile sculpture was attached to a dissolvable starch-based cloth, which was sewn and embroidered onto, including wild carrot flowering heads to represent the neuronal cell bodies. Dipping the whole sculpture into water dissolved the starch, leaving a lattice of thread and connected textiles. After drying on a mould the remaining starchy threads formed a stiff structure. This process reflects a scientific technique called CLARITY where neurons are fluorescently tagged and then the brain is 'cleared' of lipids, leaving a 3D lattice of neuronal projections, which you can image using a high-powered microscope.

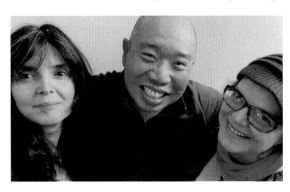

Giles Yeo is a programme leader at the MRC Metabolic Diseases Unit in Cambridge and his research currently focuses on the influence of genes on feeding behaviour and bodyweight. Jane Goodall is also a Cambridge scientist who researches the mechanism of unwanted weight loss during heart failure and its link to neurones involved in brain control of food intake. Clare Goodall is a medieval storyteller and historical costumer who worked on this unusual project with hand sewing and a sewing machine.

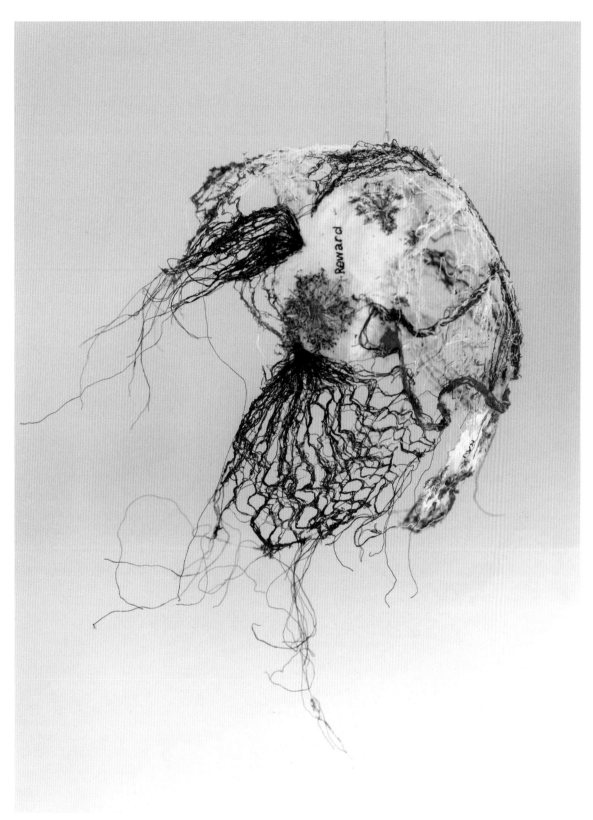

The 'Making Connections' sculpture was a collaboration between Giles Yeo and two sisters, Jane and Clare Goodall

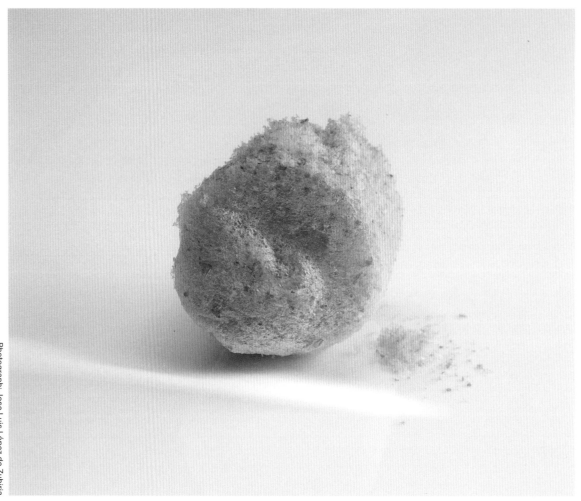

162

Andoni Luis Aduriz

CHEF

At Mugaritz we are interested in contributing to people's quality of life through gastronomy. The way in which we seek to achieve it is not only related to nutrition. We are especially interested in exploring the forces that govern our desires or our appetite. Many of our cravings are nothing more than the command of our gut to the brain when it notices the lack of certain foods.

A plate in a place like Mugaritz means many things. Sometimes it is a technical exploration, sometimes the thread of a story or even sometimes the result of an investigation. In 2014 we published *Effect of Highly Aerated Food on Expected Satiety* in the *International Journal of Gastronomy and Food Science*. That paper shows a practical way to design satiating new products by a real interaction of science and cooking. From the initial idea at Mugaritz a highly aerated product was designed to prove that the feeling of fullness starts before food is eaten, at the point when the food is just being viewed by the consumer.

Following this research, in 2016 we put it into practice within our experience. We made this flax dry meringue filled with Idiazabal cheese foam as an essay on science and health.

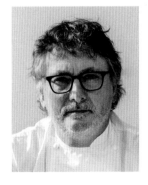

One of the most influential chefs of our times, Aduriz prioritises culinary evolution through an interdisciplinary approach. Established in 1998, his two-Michelin-starred restaurant Mugaritz, is regularly considered among the world's best and in 2021 he was rated third in the world in the Best Chef Awards. Through articles and books written alone or in collaboration with scientists and scholars, and lecturing worldwide, for example to Harvard and Tufts Universities, MIT and the Basque Culinary Center Foundation, he shares the knowledge acquired at Mugaritz – from health to the gastronomy of the future.

Dan Simpson

POET

The warmth brings me back to myself
somewhat.

I can always light a candle
and incense
and breathe
and accept the day
and accept my feelings
and accept myself
work with whatever light I have generated
even if it seems like
not quite enough.

The world outside
myself
also provides.

The moon is hidden
but still
the sky is not completely dark
and there are people
powering the streetlamps
and braking in their cars
and putting up fairy lights
so how can any of us
be alone?

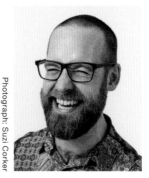

Photograph: Suzi Corker

Writer, performer, producer, and educator Dan Simpson makes highly engaging, thought-provoking, intelligent and entertaining contemporary work. His subjects include science and technology; history and place; art and culture; people and poetry. Often working in scientific contexts, he performs at popular science events and festivals worldwide. He creates pioneering work using crowdsourced and roaming poetry for organisations such as the Royal Academy of Arts, National Museum of Scotland, and the European Commission.

An enthusiastic, insightful, and adaptable workshop leader, Dan has published two collections of poetry Applied Mathematics and Totally Cultured (Burning Eye Books).

Annie Gray
FOOD HISTORIAN

My picture of health is a representation of (selected) health foods through time, from circa 1550 to around the present day. Not only does it show how attitudes to food have changed, but I hope also puts into perspective the way in which every era has its own version of exactly how you are what you eat. Things we regard as healthy and desirable now were once seen as bad, and vice versa. And things we once saw as good may have gone out of common use, and be coming round once more. Health is complex: food is complex too. All we can do is the best we can.

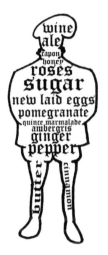
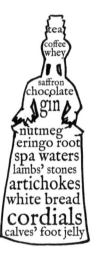
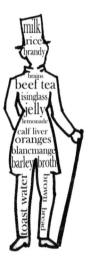
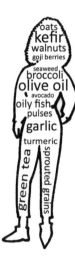

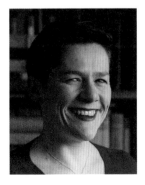

Annie Gray (PhD FRHistS) is one of Britain's leading food historians. She works as a broadcaster, author and consultant. She's a panellist on BBC Radio 4's The Kitchen Cabinet, and a TV regular. Her books include The Greedy Queen: eating with Victoria, Victory in the Kitchen: the life of *Churchill's Cook, and* At Christmas We Feast: Festive Food Through the Ages. *Annie is also a consultant for the award-winning English Heritage YouTube series,* The Victorian Way, *as well as working widely across the heritage industry. She is a research associate at the University of York.*

Amanda Fisher

MRC LMS SCIENTIST

Nobody likes to see washing up piling up in the sink at home or at work. During the first national lockdown important laboratory experiments were put on hold as clinical staff were recalled to NHS frontline duty and scientists rushed to help with national COVID-19 testing. Research laboratories struggled just to keep working. With this as a backdrop, the steady reappearance of dirty, well-used and much repaired (blue tape) glassware in laboratory sinks has become an unexpectedly joyous sight. It shows that experiments are resuming – experiments that can unleash discoveries that transform our health and the way we live. If the pandemic has taught us anything it is to reframe our views of the ordinary and mundane and most of all, to embrace Science.

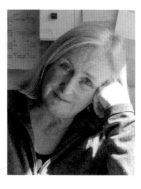

Amanda Fisher (Mandy) is a cell and molecular biologist who is particularly interested in epigenetics. She has lived and worked in France and America before joining the LMS at Imperial College London. Mandy's research looks at the interplay between genes and the environment and the impact this has for human health – a tension between nature and nurture. She has been involved in many collaborative projects exploring how scientific discoveries change the way we live, and together with Vivienne Parry in 2010, co-founded the Suffrage Science Awards to celebrate the contributions of women scientists.

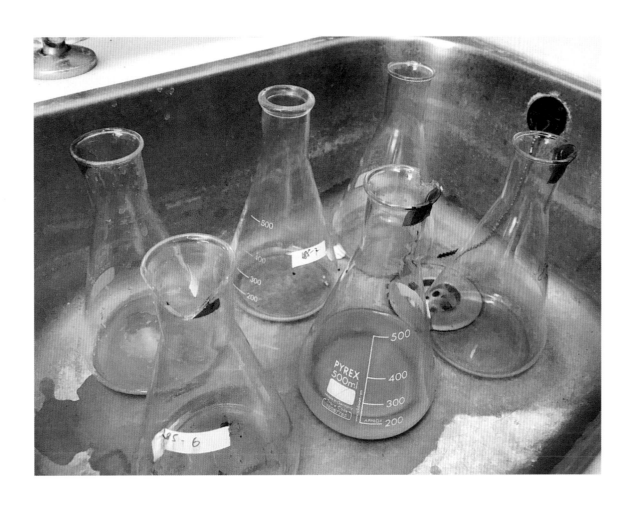

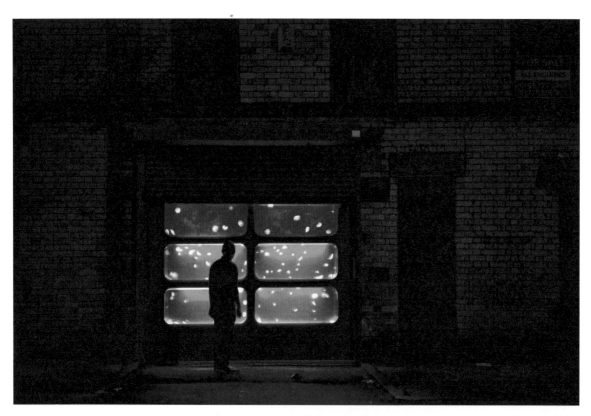

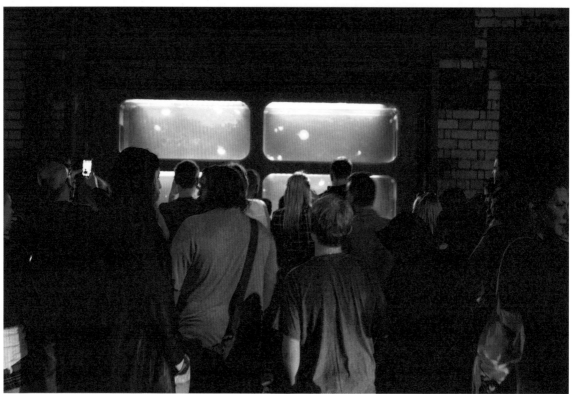

The physical possibility of inspiring imagination in the mind of somebody living.
Site specific installation, Toxteth, Liverpool during the Liverpool Biennial

Walter & Zoniel
MULTIMEDIA ARTISTS

The aim: to bring together people in a troubled area of the city by stirring their imagination. Under cover of darkness, Walter & Zoniel took over a derelict building and filled it with tanks of live jellyfish, creating the illusion that the whole building was full of the alien-like creatures.

During daytime hours the windows were covered in metal shutters, which only opened as darkness fell, to reveal the surrealist installation. Playing with the notions of inspiration and social wealth.

Revealed in absolute secrecy, with no press or PR being released about the work. The first public experience of the installation was as dusk fell, when the shutters automatically lifted to reveal the surrealism living within, allowing the artwork to affect the neighbourhood naturally. From an area of dissension and aggression people were drawn together into lively and peaceful discussion, giving us our picture of a healthy community.

The jellyfish were safely returned alive to the sea.

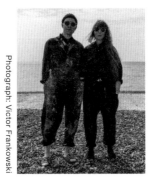

Photograph: Victor Frankowski

Raised in London, Walter would wander the concrete complexes creating installations at night, placing them publicly to be stumbled upon by day. Inspired by the workings of the universe he studied science and nebular theory before teaching himself photography. In the hills of North Wales, Zoniel's early life illness inspired a fascination with the capabilities and perception of the human mind, which she wanted to represent through art. As a teenager she moved to a Tibetan Buddhist Monastery, studying meditation and Tibetan arts. Practising as a duo since 2014, their work unites the analytical and the ethereal, merging experiences from their respective backgrounds.

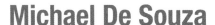

Michael De Souza
WRITER, PUBLISHER AND SWIMMING CONSULTANT

Irie is a word from a Caribbean land
It's a word from the Rastaman!
A Rastaman is a Caribbean bloke
He has a serious face, but he loves to joke.
So he created this special word.
That may seem strange or even absurd
Irie is a word that means a positive ting.
It could be food or it could be Bling.
It could be a night it could be a day!
It could be the way your football team play!
When you're feeling Irie you're feeling right
When you're feeling Irie you're
feeling brighter than bright
When you're feeling Irie you're as
happy as can be...
We all owe it to our selves to feel...
... IRIE!

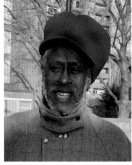

Photograph: Richard Adams

Born in Trinidad and Tobago in the mid-fifties, Michael De Souza settled in Notting Hill, London. After several years as a mechanical engineer, he answered his true calling becoming a play worker at Acklam Rd Adventure Playground. Qualifying as a football and swimming coach in 1987, he created alter ego singing swimming teacher Professor Splash, who's been entertaining and highly successful for 30 years. Encouraging swimmers using rhymes he discovered his love of writing and embarked on books about council house mouse Rastamouse, which were adapted as a very popular CBeebies animated TV series. Michael is now scripting the Rastamouse movie and putting finishing touches to his latest book introducing another lovable character Lil Bruv, a six-year-old wordsmith.

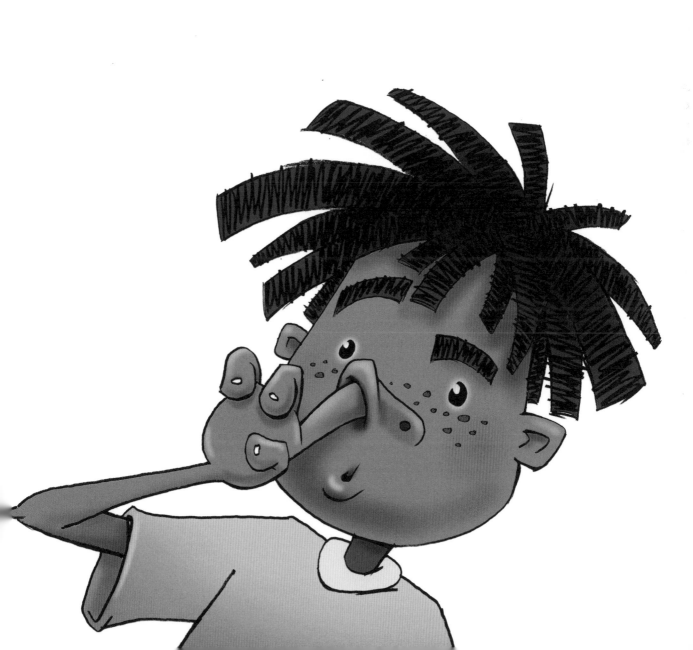

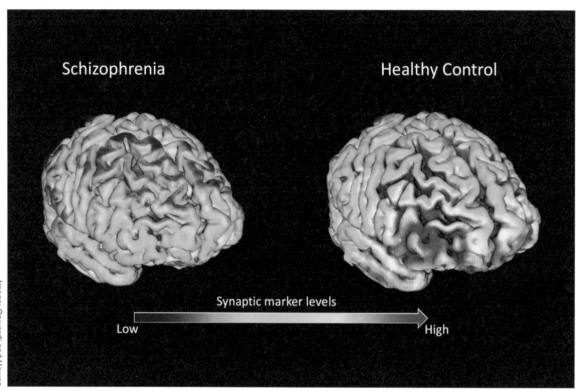

Schizophrenia

Healthy Control

Synaptic marker levels

Low

High

Oliver Howes
CLINICIAN SCIENTIST

Our brains are key to what makes us human. Communication between nerve cells in the brain underlies thinking, speaking, and behaving. Nerve cells communicate with each other through connections called synapses. These allow information to pass from one nerve cell to the next. Brains start to fail when synapses don't work efficiently or are lost, leading to mental disorders.

This image summarises findings from brain scans that measure the levels of a protein marker of the level of synapses in the brain. The scan on the left shows average levels of this protein in people with schizophrenia, whilst the one on the right shows average levels in healthy controls. The levels of the protein throughout the brain are illustrated by the colours: blue indicates low levels, whilst red high levels. People with schizophrenia show lower levels of this protein than healthy people throughout their brains, particularly in the regions at the front involved in thinking and planning behaviour. This could explain the problems people with schizophrenia have in thinking and planning, as well as other symptoms of the disorder. We are now following up on this discovery, to determine the role of this protein in the onset of the illness, and the potential to develop new treatments for the illness that prevent synapse loss.

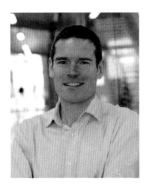

Professor of Molecular Psychiatry at King's and Imperial Colleges, London, and Consultant Psychiatrist at The Maudsley Hospital, Oliver Howes' research centres on the causes and treatment of affective and psychotic disorders. Recipient of many awards including the Royal College of Psychiatrists Researcher of the Year Award 2017, Howes was named one of the most influential researchers in the world by Web of Science in 2019. He was elected as a Fellow of the Academy of Medical Sciences in 2020. During lockdown, he got an award for the runner most likely to run downhill in his neighbourhood! He spends his spare time trying to find the world's best ice-cream.

Jane Mackay

ARTIST

I am sure that the SARS-CoV-2 pandemic has affected us in more ways than we can yet judge, both mentally as well as physically. There is no doubt that the effect of lockdown on artists forced many who work collaboratively into unaccustomed solitude. At a stroke, my previously 'healthy life' was truncated. Confined to barracks except for exercise and essential shopping, uncertainty and dejection descended. In addition to the threat of infection, friends and family were banished, travel forbidden, exhibitions cancelled, and no live music was permitted: which, for me, meant no concerts, no wind quintets, and no choral singing. What little energy remaining was diverted from creativity into confronting the many logistical complications that now beset daily existence. Not only was there no incentive to paint but the zest for life normally boosted by friends and pursuits dissipated rapidly. It was as if one was struggling through a dense, dark forest, tripping over tree roots, becoming entangled in creepers and vines, fearful of what was lurking in the shadows. Although the healing process is not yet complete, this picture of health sequence endeavours to illustrate my own journey from darkness to light. Though synaesthetic visions of music form the cornerstone of my art practice, I also experience visual images relating to psychological matters and events, and I have employed some of these in this triptych.

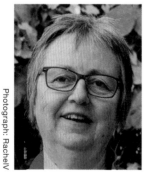

Photograph: RachelV

Jane Mackay – always a prolific painter but also intrigued by the sciences, originally studied medicine, subsequently working in Papua New Guinea, and as a GP in London. At the millennium she relinquished this career for full-time art, gaining an MFA from the University of the Arts London, in 2016. Her colourful, abstract paintings based on synaesthetic images generated by music have been exhibited widely in the UK and Europe, and featured in the press, music publications, television and film. She has recently extended the scope of her art, transcribing psychological experiences on to canvas.

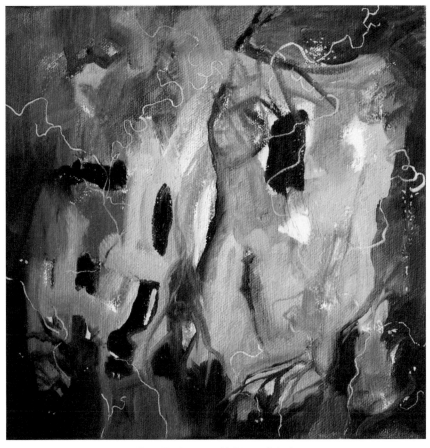

From Darkness to Light – a triptych
A representation of the gloomy jungle/forest, and the stumbling towards
the light, glimpsed as yellow-orange-pink through branches

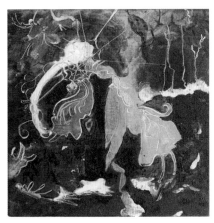

We are not out of the woods yet, but organic
life is much more apparent: roots are
sprouting, cobwebs woven, spirits stirring

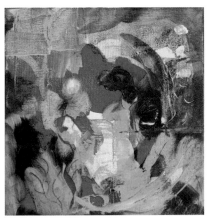

A riot of colour and movement: the shapes
now appear to be travelling through a long
tube at high speed, out of the forest and
into the light

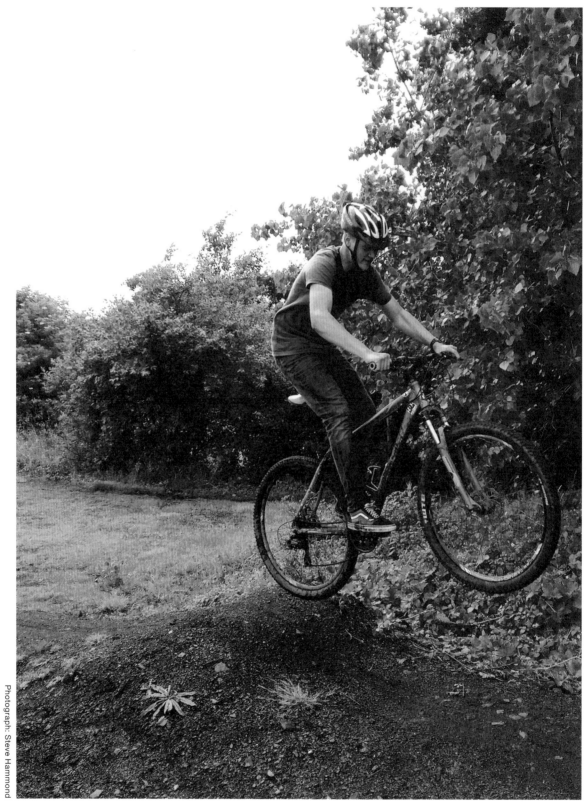

Nick Vincent

GRAPHIC DESIGNER

My picture of health is 15-year-old Ben Hammond loving riding his bike in July 2016.

Tragically the day after this picture which was taken by his father Steve, he unexpectedly died from a heart anomaly.

Every week in the UK at least 12 young people die of undiagnosed heart conditions.

Ben was about to take on a career in agriculture. He had already started working on a local dairy farm in Kent at the weekend. He was showing a real passion for arable farming and was expecting to attend agricultural college when he left school.

Steve, Sheralyn and Ben's younger brother Archie continue to show unbelievable courage every day. And together with a small group of friends they started Team Ben Hammond, a fundraising group working on behalf of Cardiac Risk in the Young. The local community have so far helped us provide 750 heart screenings for young people.

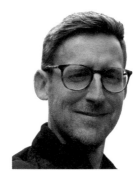

Nick has 20+ years of expertise in branding, print, campaigns, public engagement and digital. He founded Vincent Design with his partner in 2008 to work with like-minded clients in the research, not-for-profit and education sectors with a simple ambition. To design for good. He is very proud to be part of the Team Ben Hammond committee, and ran the London Marathon in 2017 and the Great North Run in 2018 for Ben.

Celine Marchbank
PHOTOGRAPHIC ARTIST

After my mother's death, I took on an allotment plot across the street from my home in South London. The plot needed much work; hours of weeding, clearing and constant maintaining proceeded and never really stopped, but in return it nurtured and cared for me too. The activities kept me healthy both physically and mentally, but most importantly it allowed me to process my grief. It made me take care of myself, its fruit and vegetable offerings nurtured and cared for me, it brought me back to life through a dark time.

I have inherited my mother's love of gardening, and all things flowers related, when I'm on my allotment I'm reminded of her and feel connected. It is a happy place for me to be, it offers calm moments within this busy city life, it's my picture of health, every time I walk through the gates I feel well again.

My photograph was made on one of my early evening strolls around the allotment, it is the flower of a Squash plant, taken in late summer as the weather turned to autumn. It is a magical time of year there, whilst most of the produce is coming to an end as the season changes, the squashes are just getting going, in a rush to reach their beautiful full potential before winter sets in. As the weather turns this sight gives me a sense of hope.

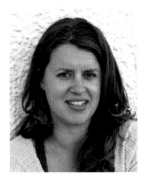

Celine Marchbank is an award-winning London-based photographic artist. Her practice explores the quiet everyday details of domesticity. Celine's first book; Tulip, *the story of the last year of her mother's life, published by Dewi Lewis in 2016, was met with widespread acclaim, named* The Observer *Photo Book of the Month and Photo-Eye Photo Book of The Week, featured in* The British Journal of Photography, *BBC News,* Vanity Fair *amongst many others. Her second book,* A Stranger in my Mother's Kitchen, *is a 5-year exploration into the grieving process told through photographs, writing and her mother's recipes.*

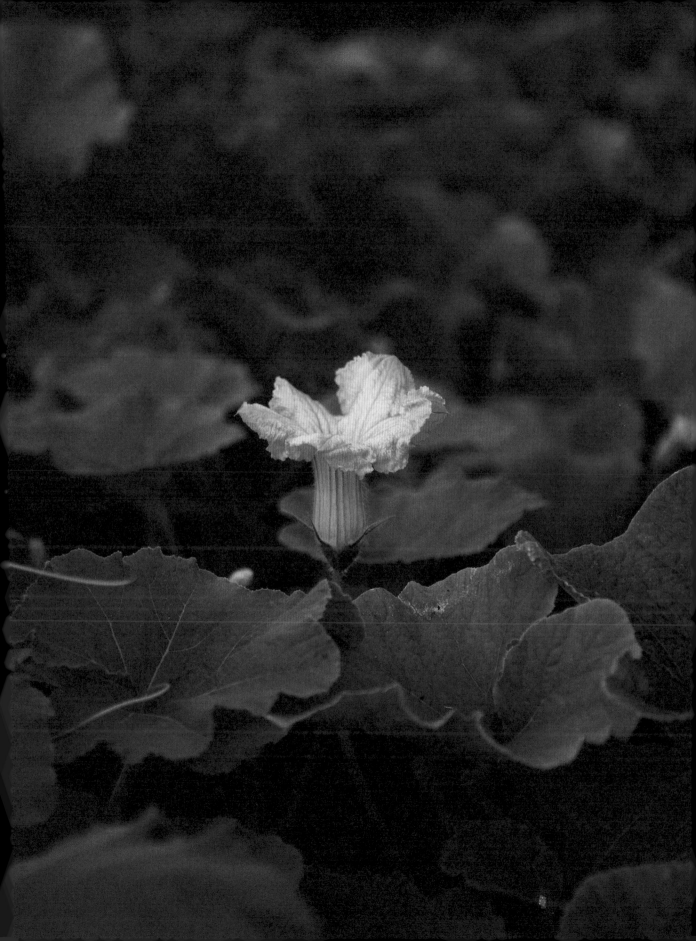

Roman Snow
PRODUCTION DESIGN STUDENT

My last visit to Palestine was in 2017 and this footage was part of my final major project at Camberwell, UAL. In this video I simply placed the camera on a coffee table and pressed record, trying to capture the soldiers routine as if I was not there. While I was not disturbed during recording the soldiers were well aware of my presence and some can be seen looking directly into the camera. I think the kids in this video are the true heroes of this performance who, in defiance of such an oppressive environment, retain their qualities as children. In the midst of conflict there is always the need to keep moving and stay healthy.

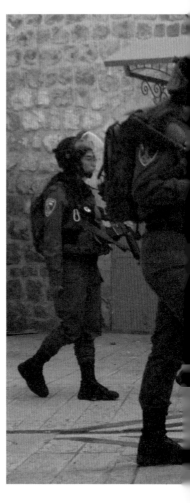

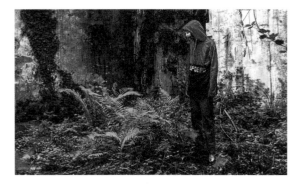

I am a set design student in the final year of my BA at University of the Arts London (UAL). Photography and video are both passions of mine and I involve myself in these activities daily trying to capture a narrative that expresses itself before me. Having a plethora of shooting locations for photography here where my family live in Italy, I find myself becoming an avid explorer; capturing with my camera relics from the Cold War and pre-mediaeval sunken churches.

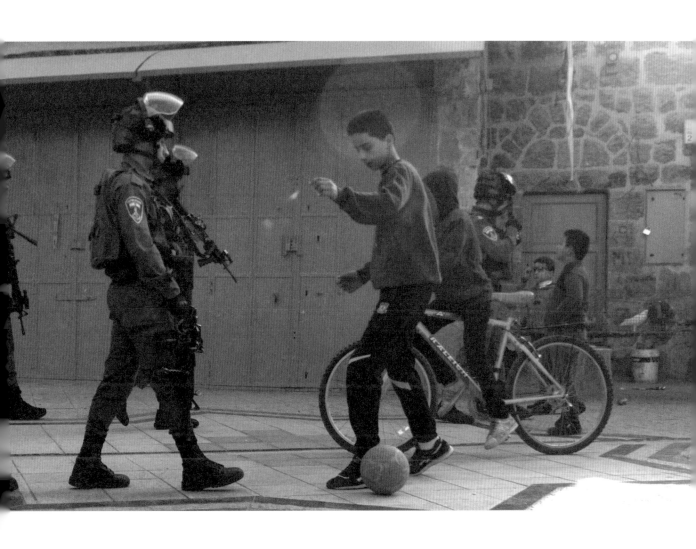

Mahmoud Alhaj

MULTIMEDIA ARTIST

Responding to the conflict in Gaza, the works from my 'Fragile' series employ empty blister sheets from various medications. Superimposed with images of buildings and open windows, the sheets themselves take on a sculptural quality and exhibit deeply rooted pain and anxiety in war-torn urban centres. Palestine has been in a military quarantine state for decades and due to the pandemic has been increasingly ignored on the global stage. For me, this intense isolation has created a need to escape reality by creating alternate worlds through found materials. In these images, I explore the use of easily accessible medication to sedate those experiencing constant distress, and imply the need for intentional mental and physical healing on a global scale.

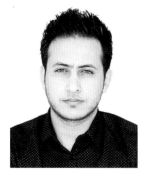

Palestinian visual artist and teacher Alhaj received a BA in Journalism and Media from Al-Aqsa University (2012) and has taught visual arts at the Palestine Red Crescent Society since 2017. In 2019, he collaborated with Dutch artist Suzanne Groothuis on a land art workshop *'Intimate Terrains' for the Palestine Museum. He has exhibited widely in Palestine, Europe and the USA, including in Art in Isolation at the Middle East Institute in Washington DC (2020); Within the Vacuum at Shababek for Contemporary Art, Palestine (2019);* *Contemplative Contrasts at the A.M. Qattan Foundation, Palestine (2019) and Orient 2.0 at Pulchri Studio, Netherlands (2017).*

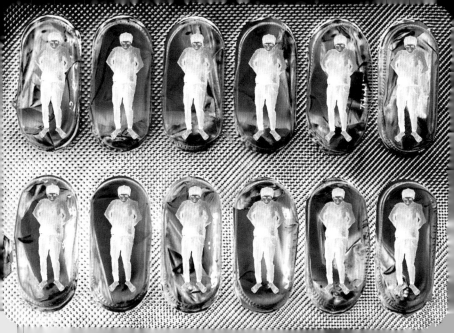

Jon Snow

JOURNALIST

I confess this is what comes to mind!
My grandson Marley who was one year old on 19th November –
I painted him in water colour that day!

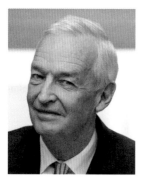

Jon Snow joined ITN in 1976 reporting from Africa, the Middle East and Europe, becoming Washington correspondent then diplomatic correspondent until 1989 when he became main anchor of Channel 4 News. He has reported on many major world events including the fall of Idi Amin; the Soviet invasion of Afghanistan; the release of Nelson Mandela, earthquakes in Kashmir and Haiti, and the election of Barack Obama, winning numerous awards including in 2015, the BAFTA Fellowship. Jon served on the boards of Britain's National Gallery and Tate Gallery, and for thirty years was chairman of New Horizon, a London day centre for homeless and vulnerable teenagers.

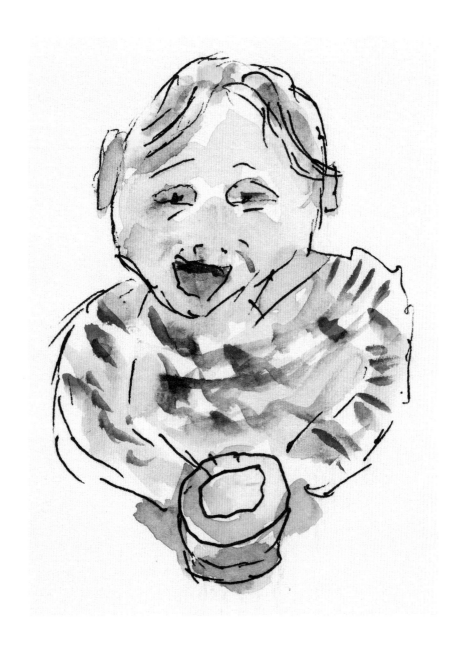

John Gurdon

DEVELOPMENTAL BIOLOGIST

This is a painting I did at school, about 60 years ago. At school we were required to give some time to art under the teaching of a well-known man at that time, called Wilfred Blunt, who later became director of an art gallery near Guildford, Surrey. For the one-hour session each week we were required to paint or draw some object which each time was different. I asked if I could be excused from that requirement and concentrate entirely on one painting which I was engaged in out of interest – a picture of butterflies that could be seen on blackberry bushes. I was more interested in spending two years doing one painting than trying to do some representation of a new object each week. The art master agreed to this.

What could this possibly have to do with *A Picture of Health*? There is no simple answer to this. Except that the preoccupation with this painting kept me in good health for one lesson per week for the last two years of my time at the school.

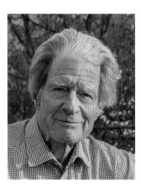

John Gurdon joined the MRC Laboratory of Molecular Biology in Cambridge in 1971 and went on, along with Professor Laskey, to co-found a research institute of developmental and cancer biology, which now shares his name: The Gurdon Institute. His research concentrates on nuclear transplantation in Xenopus, experimenting to discover the value of mRNA microinjection, and mechanisms of nuclear reprogramming. Master of Magdalene College Cambridge between 1995 and 2002, in 2009 he was awarded the Lasker Award for Basic Medical Science and in 2012, the Nobel Prize for Physiology or Medicine.

RUBUS FRUTICOSUS IN JULY.

Limenitis camilla var. nigrina

Apatura
Iris

Apatura
Iris

Limenitis
camilla

Limenitis
camilla

Argynnis
paphia

Thecla
betulae

Argynnis
cydippe

Argynnis
cydippe

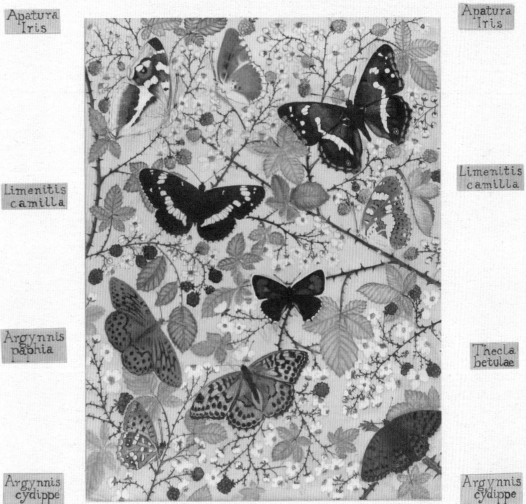

Argynnis paphia var. valezina

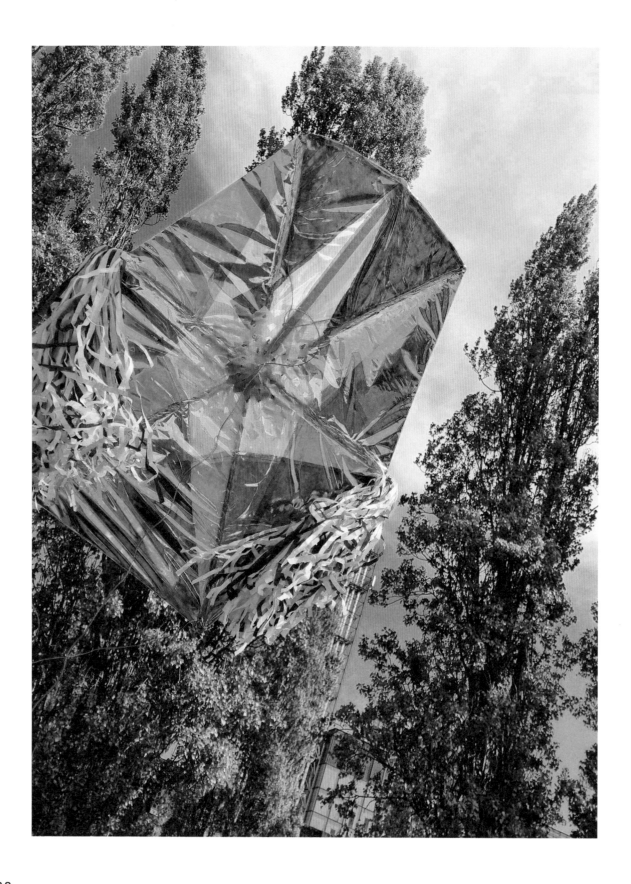

Fazil Khan

FACILITIES OFFICER, LMS

How I find my peace of mind

I was born in Guyana (South America) and when I first attended school along with all the other students we were taught how to make and fly kites. I was 5 years old at the time and the point of the kites was related to Easter and to celebrate the resurrection of Christ. This is a very important thing in Guyana. This period in my life was very enjoyable and I fondly remember the experience.

I first came to London when I was 13 and stopped making and flying kites as there was such a big culture difference.

At the age of 55 during the pandemic and the absolute lockdown I was living alone in Chelmsford and my family were a long way away in a different part of London where I used to live. We are a close knit family and I missed that. Also, where I am the local pub is central to the community where everyone knows each other. The landlord often used to organise trips out for the locals such as night meetings at Chelmsford racecourse. When these situations stopped because of lockdown I took up making kites again and after restrictions lifted I passed on my skills to the children of my friends.

I go to many kite festivals and love it again. We have all been affected by COVID in one way or another and find our own way out, and when flying my kites no matter how many other flyers or spectators, I feel I am the only one there focusing on the kite, controlling it. There is just me and the sound of the breeze.

Fazil Khan, or Faz for short, has been at the LMS for 12 years working in the Estates and Facilities team where he supports the Institute's activities by covering goods deliveries and health and safety issues for some of the labs. Before this he worked for the courts and is described by friends and colleagues as a 'man of fashion and dance'.

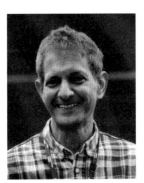

189

Susan Simon
MRC DIRECTOR CAPITAL & ESTATES

This picture has been carved in leather and painted with dye and acrylics. It is inspired by the photograph 'Eating for Two' of the innards of a female fruit fly found in the LMS's BPoD extensive archive of beautiful images (August 2015), originating from research at the LMS by Irene Miguel-Aliaga's group. It has always fascinated me and represents my amazement over the work of scientists and the beauty of nature, which extends well beyond what the naked eye can see.

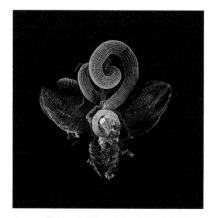

Image: Tobias Reiff et al, in *eLife*, July 2015

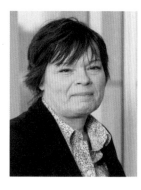

I was born in Leipzig and grew up in East-Germany (GDR), attended state school and qualified as a commercial clerk eventually landing in the construction industry as a project manager. With the move to the UK in 2010, I took every opportunity to study, which was not open to me in East Germany and since then completed a Masters in Business and Administration, Masters in Construction Law and a Doctorate in Business and Administration. I have been employed by the MRC since 2010 and had the privilege to work with many of our scientists and operational staff creating new research facilities or improving existing ones.

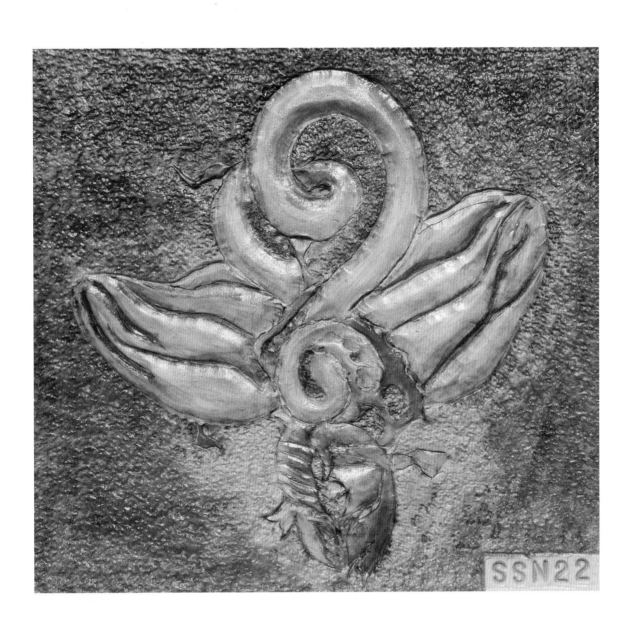

SSN22

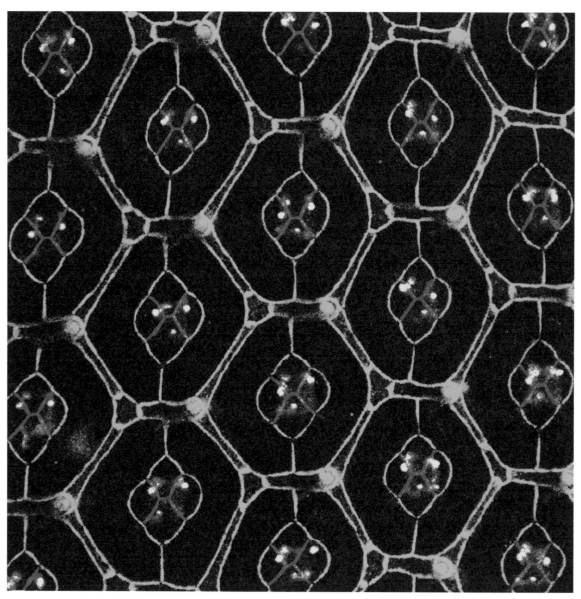

Image by Eunice HoYee Chan et al, in *eLife*, May 2017

Lux Fatimathas
SCIENCE WRITER

This image inspired the design etched into the glass and cladding of the new LMS building – its outer skin. It shows a picture of cells linked to their neighbours via proteins called cadherins. These cadherins attach to flexible scaffolds within cells and enable them to contort themselves into different shapes. Researchers have begun investigating how cadherins affect the shape of cells within the eyes of fruit flies, in order to get a better handle of how our own cells form all the different tissues in the human body. The decorative pattern that wraps around the new LMS building, is part of the growing collection in the LMS's beautiful BPoD archive, giving a daily update on scientific and health discoveries that capture our imagination.

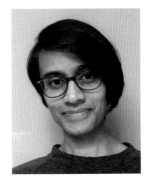

Lux Fatimathas is a science and healthcare writer, with a BSc in neuroscience and a PhD in cell and molecular biology from University College London. Leaving a career as a lab scientist behind, she moved into science communications while working for the National University of Singapore and has also worked in science publishing. Today she is a freelance writer in London, covering a breadth of health and biomedical topics.

Wormwood Scrubs Pony Centre

EQUINE THERAPY CENTRE FOR CHILDREN

This picture shows a thriving scene at the Wormwood Scrubs Pony Centre where children and ponies are enjoying the fun of being together in a safe outdoor venue where they can also receive lots of fresh air.

The ponies give opportunities for the children to be joyful. Whilst at the centre the young people and volunteers will be taking plenty of healthy physical exercise. Many life skills can also be developed and learnt. All this is carried out in a caring and supportive environment. The ponies become the catalyst to learning and they can change lives for the better for all those who may spend time with them. Valuable time spent in the company of a pony can also lead to developing confidence and friendships.

The Pony Centre is a place where people with physical disabilities or learning difficulties are made welcome. People with dementia can come to stroke a pony. This often results in bringing a smile of happiness onto their faces.

Wormwood Scrubs Pony Centre is certainly a beautiful, living picture of health that is very much needed in today's society.

Founded by Mary Joy Langdon in 1989, the Wormwood Scrubs Pony Centre has hosted thousands of children and adult volunteers, and all have been enriched by their time spent at this little rural oasis situated in West London. Recipient of The Queen's Award for Voluntary Service – equivalent of the MBE and the highest award that can be made to a voluntary group – the centre is a registered charity, a Riding for the Disabled Association member, and offers the British Horse Society 'Changing Lives Through Horses' programme. All the activities at the centre can greatly help young people to have better mental and physical health.

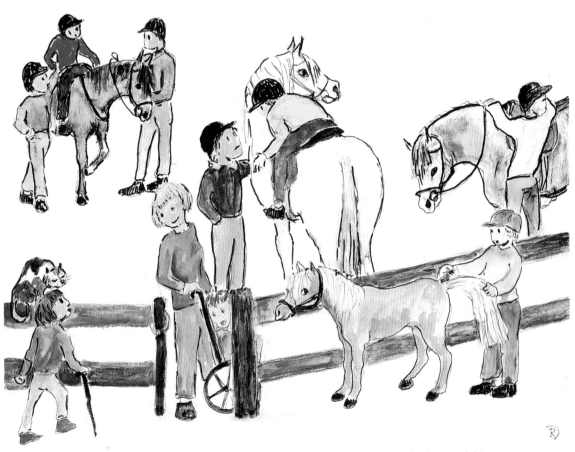

Drawing: Romaine Dennistoun. Working from life in pen, ink and watercolours, for the past eight years Romaine Dennistoun has been Artist in Residence at the Wormwood Scrubs Pony Centre

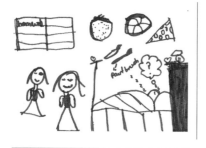

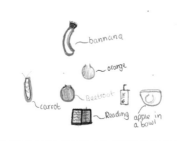

- bannana
- orange
- carrot
- Beetroot
- Reading
- apple in a bowl

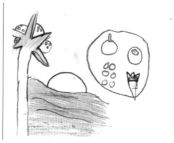

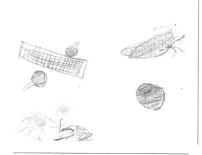

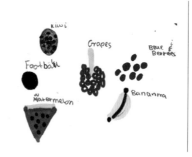

Kiwi

Football

Grapes

Blue & Berries

Watermelon

Bananna

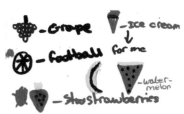

- Grape
- Ice cream
- football   for me
- water-melon
- Stra Strawberries

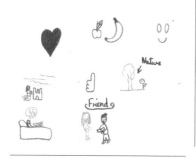

Nature

Friend

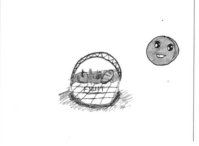

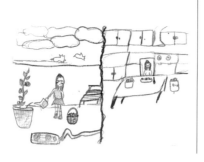

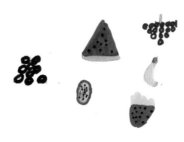

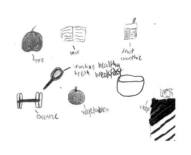

Apple

book

fruit smoothie

brushing teeth

healthy breakfast

exercise

vegetables

sleep

ReachOut

MENTORING CHARITY

These pictures were drawn by a group of 10- and 11-year-old girls who take part in a mentoring programme for underserved young people in London. Scientists from the LMS delivered a workshop to the students that encouraged them to be curious and ask questions about the world around us – "that's what makes a good scientist" they were told. It was very inspiring coming from a young Indian female scientist who was a role model to them. The girls in turn were asked what they think of when they hear the phrase *A Picture of Health*. Many drew fruit, or depicted exercise, sleep and nature – all key components of a healthy lifestyle. Some drew experiences as their picture of health such as building a sandcastle, being with friends, gardening and reading. And one girl drew a scene from the Caribbean island where she's from – a palm tree on the beach at sunset.

ReachOut is a mentoring charity that gives amazing young people from economically disadvantaged communities in London weekly one-to-one support from a volunteer mentor. We help them to develop their character, raise aspirations and improve their academic attainment through long-term one-to-one mentoring to help them achieve their potential and go on to lead good, happy and successful lives.

Brian Patten

POET

A Peach for Linda

Dear heart,
I've found a special cannula into which
Our future's pumped.
Warm evenings drip into the blood,
The scent of fig trees too,
And in between each drop
Winds a dusty path that leads
To a tavern on the beach
Where all we ever wanted
Is still within our reach,
And where we can order wine
And share a peach.

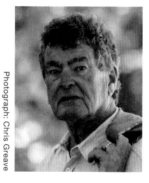

Brian Patten was born in Liverpool and rose to fame with Penguin's seminal The Mersey Sound collection (1967), now a Penguin Modern Classic. His publications include Collected Love Poems (Harper Perennial) and Selected Poems (Penguin Books), and for children, Beowulf Monster Slayer (Barrington Stoke 2020). Patten is a master performer of his work and has read in venues as varied as the Queen Elizabeth Hall in London and the Students Union in Khartoum. His most recent book is The Book of Upside Down Thinking, comic verse inspired by traditional stories from the Near and Middle East.

Juan-Ángel Vicente Bravo

BEE KEEPER

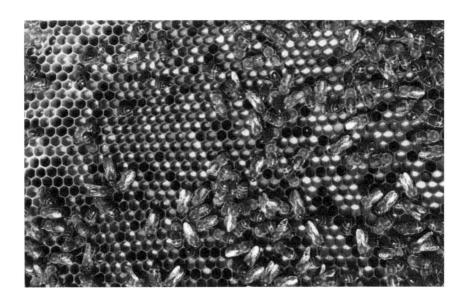

This is a picture of health because after a long and very dry winter, with the hive barely surviving due to lack of food and the dreaded varroa (the parasite which is becoming an ever increasing threat to the health of honeybees), the spring has begun with a great explosion of flowers providing essential reserves for the hive.

Here we see worker bees free of varroa and looking healthy as they store nectar and pollen in the honeycomb. In two or three days, the queen bee will fill the honeycomb with eggs, thus assuring the future of the hive for this year.

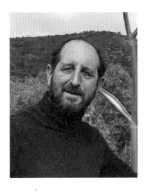

I have been a professional beekeeper for 22 years in the region of Extremadura in South West Spain. I am an experienced beekeeper, but against the backdrop of disease (especially varroa) and the consequences of climate change (prolonged drought and the lack of adequate food sources),

I can see that there is a progressive decline in the health of honeybees and their hives which I fear could ultimately lead to their destruction.

199

Sarah Gavron
FILM DIRECTOR

This photo is of a group of young people in an Afrobeats dance class. The team was inspired to create this scene, for our collaborative film *Rocks*, after we had seen similar dance and choir classes that were held at the youth club Platform, in North London. The classes were always so full of joy and laughter and keenly attended by local young people. Safe spaces for young people are now more vital than ever, for maintaining physical and mental health.

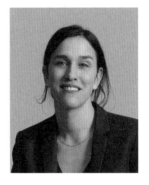

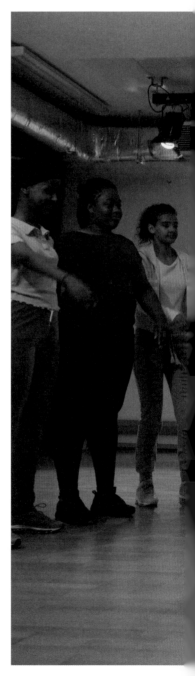

Sarah Gavron directed the recent film Rocks *in collaboration with the creative team and cast.* Rocks *was nominated for seven BAFTAs and won best British film at the British Independent film awards. In 2015* Suffragette, *directed by Sarah, opened the London Film Festival.*

Her first feature film was Brick Lane. *Prior to this, Sarah's first full-length drama,* This Little Life *for BBC TV, won the Dennis Potter award. Sarah's feature documentary,* The Village at the End of the World *in 2013, was nominated for The Grierson Award and won the Margaret*

Mead Award. In her early career, Sarah worked on documentaries for the BBC and Channel Four.

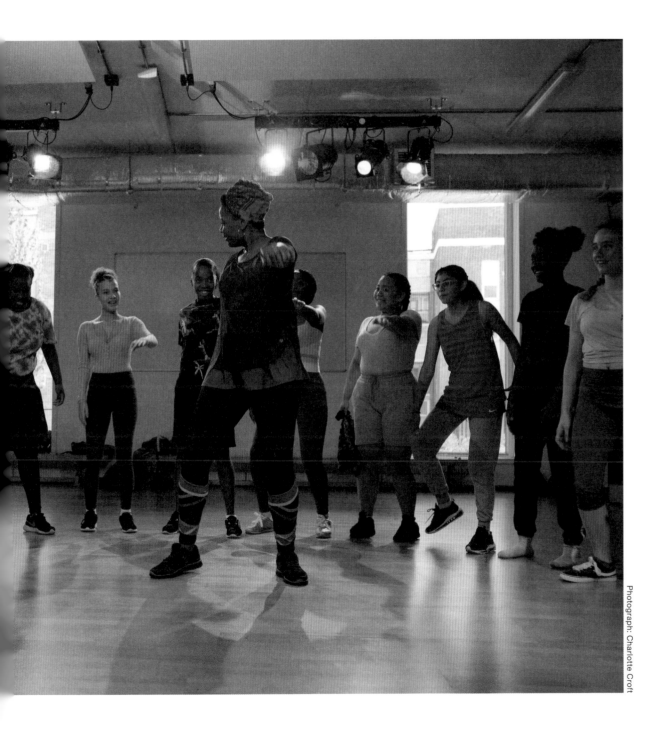

Photograph: Charlotte Croft

Charlie Phillips
PHOTOGRAPHER

I took this photograph at the 1967 Notting Hill Carnival, the first having been held the year before, and called the Notting Hill Festival. It started out as a children's carnival since they were the main focus, but when people heard the steelpan and the noisy procession people poured out of their houses and within a short time there were about two or three hundred people on the streets. The festival founder, Mrs Rhaune Laslett, used to rent a flat-bed truck and the children would be shoved on the back wearing wildly colourful costumes their parents made using feathers, paper and fabric remnants, whatever came to hand.

This photograph was taken overlooking Acklam Road which runs parallel with the Westway, an overhead stretch of motorway running from Shepherd's Bush to Paddington and a focal point of local discontent when a vast area of social housing was demolished to make way for its construction in the late 1960s.

Together with Acklam Road, All Saints Road was the beating heart of the Notting Hill Carnival and The Mangrove Restaurant the place where steel bands would gather and play along the length of the street throughout the Bank Holiday weekend. The street was also a judging point where Carnival Kings and Queens would compete, overloaded floats paraded, and towering sound systems were strategically set up in shop doorways, which would become a major feature of what became an annual event.

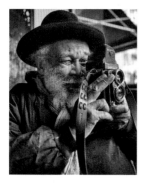

Ronald 'Charlie' Phillips, OBE, nicknamed Smokey, is a Jamaican-born restaurateur, photographer and documenter of Black London, now best known for his photographs of Notting Hill in the sixties. As a youngster working in his parents' restaurant in the Portobello road, *he was given a Kodak Retinette by a black American serviceman, so his career began accidentally when he started by photographing life in Notting Hill. Later he covered a variety of subjects, and his work has been exhibited internationally. He has published two widely* *acclaimed books: 'Notting Hill in the Sixties', 1991; 'How Great Thou Art: 50 Years of African Caribbean Funerals in London', 2014.*

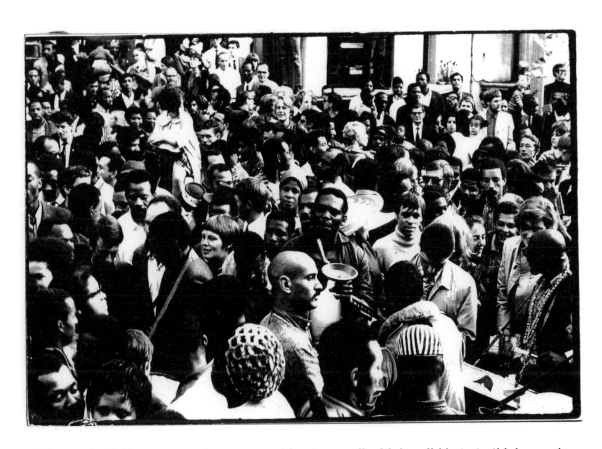

Rhaune Laslett was a good woman and I got on well with her. I'd hate to think people have left her out of the history of carnival because of her colour. I never went on the streets playing for anyone before I did it for her. I'd never done that before and I had the only steel band at the time. The first time I did the rounds through Notting Hill was the day I did it for Mrs Laslett. Carnival started with her. If anyone can tell me the name of anyone who played before that I'd be very curious.

JAZZ PIANIST, RUSS HENDERSON, MBE

William Rankin

EUROPEAN AUTHOR AND ILLUSTRATOR

Born in Edinburgh, William attended Glasgow School of Art and West of England College of Art. He is a winner of the Observer Young Cartoonist of the Year. He has authored award winning books and his drawings have been published around the world, in publications including Oz, Nova, the Radio Times *and* Actuel. *Most widespread is his Puma logo. In Paris, he was art director and Director of Internet Services of the* International Herald Tribune. *Currently underway is a book with a fresh view of the Dreyfus Affair, and a biography of the Swedish taxonomist Linnaeus.*

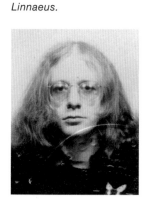

Were you to examine the crest of the British Medical Association you might notice that the supporting figure representing Hippocrates is clutching a pomegranate.

The same fruit features in the arms of Royal College of Midwives, The Royal College of Obstetricians and Gynaecologists, The Royal College of Physicians, Medical Society of London and Royal College of Physicians and Surgeons of Glasgow...

That the pomegranate features so widely speaks to its prized medicinal properties. In the first century the Greek physician and botanist Dioscorides recorded that the pomegranate could cure ulcers, earache, grief in the nostrils and expel tapeworm.

Just as importantly, symbolically, for the ancient Greeks, it was part of the central fertility cult mediating Persephone's life-bringing yearly return from the underworld bringing on spring.

The pomegranate figures in many religions, in Christian iconography it represents fecundity. For Buddhists, it is one of the three blessed fruits.

In Japan it is to be seen in the right hand of the goddess Kishimojin | (鬼子母神). Its myriad seeds betokening fertility. She; mother of a thousand children, goddess of easy delivery, family harmony, love, well-being and safety.

It was precisely in this spirit that the facing watercolour was painted for a dear Japanese friend who had her heart set on having a baby.

Prayers were answered, she was blessed with a girl.

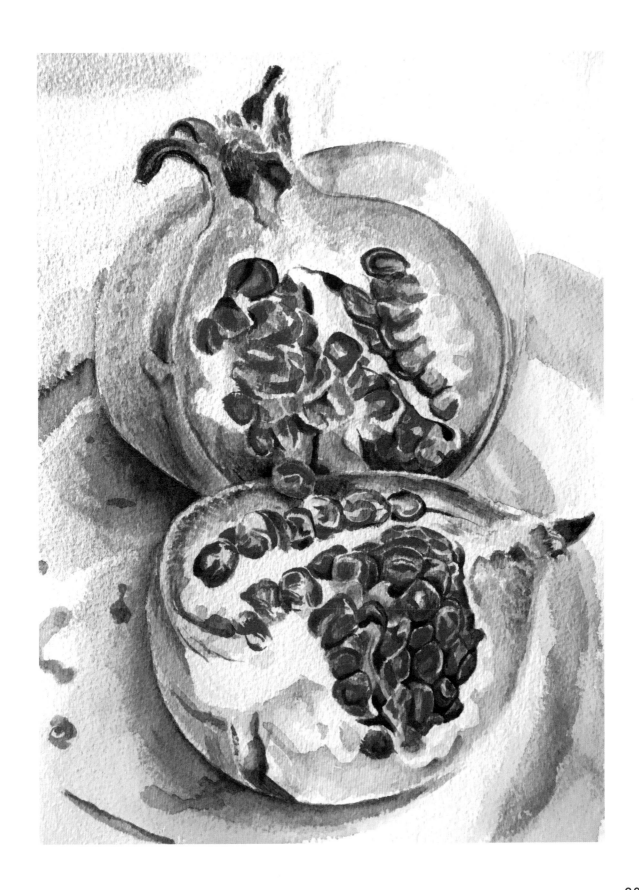

Veronika Shoot

CLASSICAL PIANIST AND YOGA TEACHER

I believe I am an alchemist in training, that is where the drive comes from. Growing up surrounded by nature and creatives of all walks of life has given me some of the foundations that drive my passion to expand the horizons of musical sharing in a way that stimulates personal connection and bold expression in innovative ways, and away from an accustomed stage. I enjoy working on numerous collaborative projects, combining music, film, storytelling, and movement. I love to create and transmute what is already present into new forms, in music, in life, in sharing and support others in that. My picture of health and sound of health comes from my passion for the devotional aspect of sound in a way that is not aiming for perfectionism but simply devoted to something other than the self. I have experienced the healing aspects of sound and mantra chanting in myself and others, due to the vibration produced from the sound and particular resonance of the Sanskrit language. This is why I wanted to share the love mantra Tumi Bhaja re Mana.

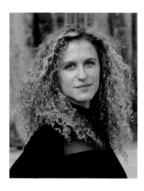

Born in Moscow and brought up in the UK, I am a classically trained pianist and also a qualified yoga teacher (I did my training in India) and have developed a yoga class specially for musicians that I run once a week. I am passionate about sharing music in a way that inspires a feeling of participation and of healing and growth as I believe it has that power. This is why I have also devised concerts and workshops away from traditional stage in all sorts of venues. Coming from a musical family, my father being a wonderful composer I have also pioneered new music and I also write my own music.

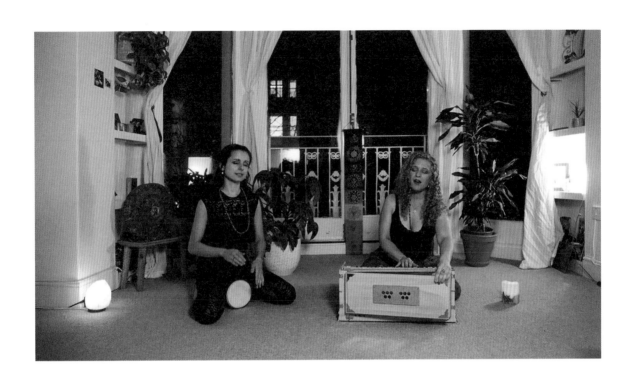

Caroline Dean and Rea Antoniou-Kourounioti

PLANT SCIENTIST AND MATHEMATICAL BIOLOGIST

Accurate timing of flowering is vital for plant species to thrive, so plants monitor seasonal cues to align flowering with spring or summer. Both daylength and temperature are similar between autumn and spring. To distinguish between these, plants have evolved what is called 'vernalization'. They first need to experience winter before they respond to 'spring-like' conditions, to flower.

In the model plant *Arabidopsis thaliana* and its relatives (e.g., broccoli, oilseed rape), vernalization is controlled by the gene *FLOWERING LOCUS C* (*FLC*). *FLC* expression changes according to the seasons. In the autumn FLC is high and prevents the plant from flowering. Over winter *FLC* is gradually silenced by an epigenetic process so that it remains stably silenced after the cold, in spring. Another gene is necessary to ensure the epigenetic silencing of *FLC*, the cold-induced *VERNALIZATION INSENSITIVE 3* (*VIN3*). *VIN3* is very low in warm conditions but it slowly increases in the cold by a process depending on the plant's reduced growth rate. These two genes respond to temperature, and especially its high and low daily fluctuations, with warm spikes repressing *VIN3* and cold nights repressing *FLC*.

Temperature fluctuations are likely to increase with climate change, which could lead to incorrect flowering time. This could be devastating for plant health, synchrony with pollinator life cycles and for agriculture because the harvested parts (e.g., fruit, seed) often depend on flowering.

Professor Dame Caroline Dean and her team dissect how plants respond to and remember winter cold. Her work focuses on a key gene that is epigenetically regulated and holds memory of the environment the plants have experienced. She is a Royal Society Professor at the John Innes Centre in Norwich and has made outstanding contributions to science and won numerous awards.

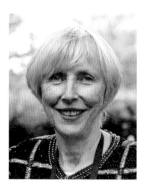

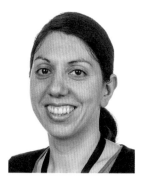

Dr Rea Antoniou-Kourounioti has been working to understand how plants extract seasonal information from fluctuating natural temperatures. Her work combines mathematical modelling and experiments in field and lab conditions. Rea is a postdoc with Caroline and Professor Martin Howard at the John Innes Centre in Norwich.

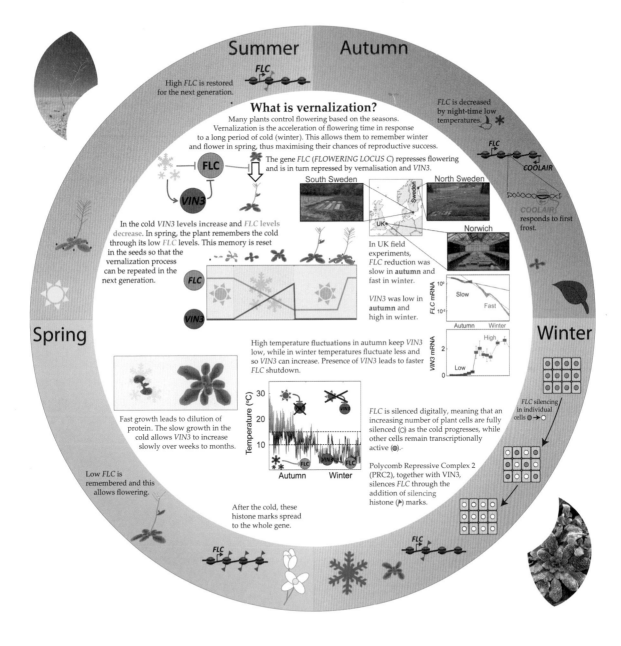

Summer   Autumn

High *FLC* is restored for the next generation.

What is vernalization?

Many plants control flowering based on the seasons. Vernalization is the acceleration of flowering time in response to a long period of cold (winter). This allows them to remember winter and flower in spring, thus maximising their chances of reproductive success.

The gene *FLC* (*FLOWERING LOCUS C*) represses flowering and is in turn repressed by vernalisation and *VIN3*.

In the cold *VIN3* levels increase and *FLC* levels decrease. In spring, the plant remembers the cold through its low *FLC* levels. This memory is reset in the seeds so that the vernalization process can be repeated in the next generation.

FLC is decreased by night-time low temperatures.

COOLAIR

COOLAIR responds to first frost.

South Sweden

North Sweden

Norwich

In UK field experiments, *FLC* reduction was slow in **autumn** and fast in winter.

VIN3 was low in **autumn** and high in winter.

FLC mRNA

Slow

Fast

Autumn   Winter

VIN3 mRNA

High

Low

Autumn   Winter

Spring   Winter

High temperature fluctuations in autumn keep *VIN3* low, while in winter temperatures fluctuate less and so *VIN3* can increase. Presence of *VIN3* leads to faster *FLC* shutdown.

Fast growth leads to dilution of protein. The slow growth in the cold allows *VIN3* to increase slowly over weeks to months.

Temperature (°C)

30
20
10

Autumn   Winter

FLC is silenced digitally, meaning that an increasing number of plant cells are fully silenced (○) as the cold progresses, while other cells remain transcriptionally active (●).

Polycomb Repressive Complex 2 (PRC2), together with VIN3, silences *FLC* through the addition of silencing histone (▶) marks.

FLC silencing in individual cells ● → ○

Low *FLC* is remembered and this allows flowering.

After the cold, these histone marks spread to the whole gene.

FLC

209

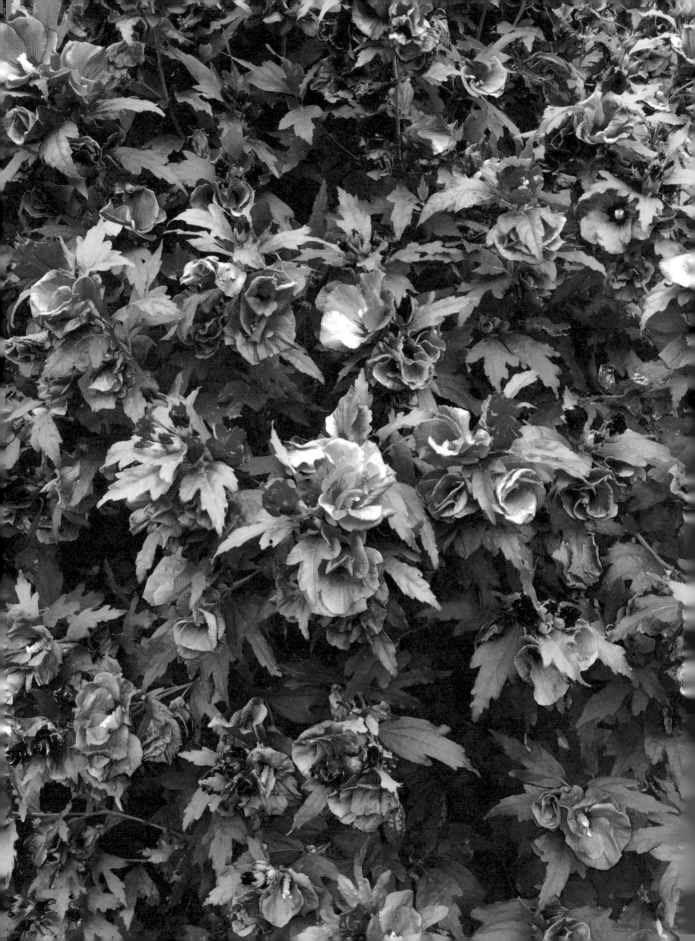

Patrick Vallance

GOVERNMENT CHIEF SCIENTIFIC ADVISER

This hibiscus in our garden shows flowers at different stages, from bud through full bloom to fading.

Its mix of colours and stages of life is what makes it beautiful. It reminded me of how much the outdoors and nature was such an important respite and tonic during the long months of the pandemic somewhere to relax, unwind, clear the mind.

Various parts of the hibiscus plant have been used in many cultures as a traditional medicine and the colour of this one has another link with medicine. William Perkin was 18 years old in 1856 and working as a chemist trying to synthesise quinine for malaria when he accidently discovered a purple dye, that he named 'mauvine'. This made his fortune as it enabled cloth to be dyed in what was then a popular but expensive colour. His factories also became the origins of the chemicals industry, which in turn helped spawn the pharmaceutical industry.

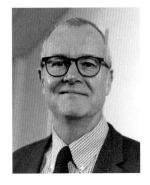

Sir Patrick Vallance is Government Chief Scientific Adviser, National Technology Adviser and Head of the Government Science and Engineering Profession. Joining in 2006, he served as president of Glaxo Smith Kline (GSK) from 2012–2017. During that time 14 new medicines for diseases ranging from cancer to HIV were approved for use worldwide. Prior to GSK, as Professor of Medicine at University College London, he led the Division of Medicine and was a consultant physician in the NHS. He is a member of the Academy of Medical Sciences and Fellow of the Royal Society.

Contributors

Acknowledgements

In 2016 the LMS was awarded funding by the UK government to build a new research home at the world-famous Hammersmith Hospital. The site in West London boasts a remarkable history of pioneering experimental medicine[1] and lies adjacent to a new landmark Biomedical Campus of Imperial College London.

Optimistic to continue making breakthroughs that improve human health, LMS researchers and their partners began *A Picture of Health* as a project to celebrate the birth of their new building and begin a collection of contemporary views on health and discovery.

A small energetic team helped to advance the project from the merest 'twinkle' in the eye towards completion. Particular thanks go to the project's curator, Lindsey Goff and the curating and events team, Kirstin von Glasow and Andree Molyneux. We thank Susan Watts, Carole Swan, Jay Stone, Jenna Stevens-Smith and members of the LMS Grants, Engagement and Communications Team, past and present, for their invaluable support and advice. Translating more than one hundred images and individual texts into a beautifully collated collection of perspectives, required the considerable artistry and skill of book designers Richard and Sam Adams, and the designer of the website, George Snow. We also thank Northend Printers, Sheffield for producing the book, and Ellie Cawthera for her lead on educational outreach at the LMS.

A Picture of Health was enabled by a pilot collaborative study between scientists and artists, co-hosted by the LMS and Central St Martins University of the Arts London (UAL) in 2019[2]. New digital content behind some of the images and stories featured in *A Picture of Health*, generated by Anthony Lewis, will become available from January 2023 onwards at lms.mrc.ac.uk/picture-of-health.

We are immensely grateful to the MRC, UKRI, Imperial College London and Walter Lilley for their sponsorship and continued enthusiasm to document the views of those within the community which the LMS serves. We also acknowledge colleagues within the MRC, LMS and UAL, too numerous to mention individually, who have been critical in shaping this project throughout its gestation.

Finally, and most importantly, we want to heartily thank all the contributors for their creative, colourful and sometimes challenging views of what *A Picture of Health* means to each of us.

Professor Dame Amanda Fisher

[1] Christopher C Booth, Medical Science and Technology at the Royal Postgraduate Medical School: the first 50 years. *British Medical Journal* 1985; : 1771–1779.

[2] apictureofhealthco.wixsite.com/about